Milestones in Drug Therapy
MDT

HMG-CoA Reductase Inhibitors

Edited by G. Schmitz and M. Torzewski

Springer Basel AG

Editors
Gerd Schmitz
Institute for Clinical Chemistry
and Laboratory Medicine
University Regensburg
Franz-Josef-Strauss-Allee 11
D-93053 Regensburg
Germany

Michael Torzewski
Johannes Gutenberg-Universität Mainz
Klinikum
Institut für Klinische Chemie und
Laboratoriumsmedizin
D-55101 Mainz
Germany

Library of Congress Cataloging-in-Publication Data
HMG-CoA reductase inhibitors / G. Schmitz, M. Torzewski, editors.
p. cm. -- (Milestones in drug therapy)
Includes bibliographical references and index.

1. Statins (Carduiovascular agents) 2. Hypercholesteremia—Chemotherapy
3. Hydroxymethylglutaryl coenzyme A reductases. I. Schmitz, G. (Gerd), 1949-
II. Torzewski, M. (Michael) III. series.

RM666.S714 H54 2002
615'.718--dc21 2002071240

Deutsche Bibliothek Cataloging-in-Publication Data
HMG-CoA reductase inhibitors / ed. by G. Schmitz and M. Torzewski. - Basel ; Boston ; Berlin: Birkhäuser, 2002
(Milestones in drug therapy)
ISBN 978-3-0348-9451-7 ISBN 978-3-0348-8135-7 (eBook)
DOI 10.1007/978-3-0348-8135-7

Originally published Birkhäuser Verlag, Basel, Switzerland in 2002

Member of the BertelsmannSpringer Publishing Group
Printed on acid-free paper produced from chlorine-free pulp. TCF ∞
Cover illustration: Potential targets for cholesterol synthesis blockers in monocyte differentiation (detail).

9 8 7 6 5 4 3 2 1 www.birkhauser-science.com

Contents

List of contributors

Stefano Bellosta, Department of Pharmacological Sciences, University of Milan, via Balzaretti 9, 20133 Milan, Italy; e-mail: Stefano.Bellosta@unimi.it

Margaret E. Brousseau, Lipid Metabolism Laboratory, Jean Mayer-USDA Human Nutrition Research Center on Aging, Tufts University, and Lipid Research Laboratory, Division of Endocrinology, Metabolism, Diabetes and Molecular Medicine, New England Medical Center, 711 Washington Street, Boston, MA 02111, USA; e-mail: mbrousseau@hnrc.tufts.edu

Alberto Corsini, Department of Pharmacological Sciences, University of Milan, via Balzaretti 9, 20133 Milan, Italy; e-mail: Alberto.Corsini@unimi.it

Colin Berry, Department of Cardiology, Western Infirmary, Glasgow G11 6NT, Scotland, UK; e-mail: colin.berry@clinmed.gla.ac.uk

Andrew Davie, Southern General Hospital, 1345 Govan Road, Glasgow G51 4TF, Scotland, UK

Helena K. Gylling, Department of Clinical Nutrition, University of Kuopio and Kuopio University Hospital, P.O. Box 1627, 70211 Kuopio, Finland; e-mail: Helena.Gylling@uku.fi

Jörg Kotzka, Abteilung Klinische Biochemie und Pathobiochemie, Deutsches Diabetes-Forschungsinstitut an der Heinrich-Heine-Universität Düsseldorf, Auf'm Hennekamp 65, 40225 Düsseldorf, Germany; e-mail: joerg.kotzka@ddfi.uni-duesseldorf.de

Wilhelm Krone, Klinik II und Poliklinik für Innere Medizin der Universität zu Köln, 50924 Köln, Germany

James K. Liao, Department of Medicine, Brigham & Women's Hospital and Harvard Medical School, 65 Landsdowne Street, Cambridge, Massachusetts 02139, USA; e-mail: jliao@rics.bwh.harvard.edu

Tatu A. Miettinen, Division of Internal Medicine, Department of Medicine, University of Helsinki, P.O. Box 340, Helsinki, FIN-00029 HUS, Finland; e-mail: tatu.a.miettinen@helsinki.fi

Dirk Müller-Wieland, Abteilung Klinische Biochemie und Pathobiochemie, Deutsches Diabetes-Forschungsinstitut an der Heinrich-Heine-Universität Düsseldorf, Auf'm Hennekamp 65, 40225 Düsseldorf, Germany; e-mail: mueller-wieland@ddfi.uni-duesseldorf.de

John McMurray, Department of Cardiology, Western Infirmary, Glasgow G11 6NT, Scotland, UK

Koichi Node, Department of Internal Medicine and Therapeutics, Osaka University Graduate School of Medicine, 2-2, Yamadaoka, Suita, Osaka 565-0871, Japan; e-mail: node@medone.med.osaka-u.ac.jp

Rodolfo Paoletti, Department of Pharmacological Sciences, University of Milan, via Balzaretti 9, 20133 Milan, Italy; e-mail: Rodolfo.Paoletti@unimi.it

Ernst J. Schaefer, Lipid Metabolism Laboratory, Jean Mayer-USDA Human Nutrition Research Center on Aging, Tufts University, and Lipid Research Laboratory, Division of Endocrinology, Metabolism, Diabetes and Molecular Medicine, New England Medical Center, 711 Washington Street, Boston, MA 02111, USA; e-mail: eschaefer@hnrc.tufts.edu

Gerd Schmitz, Institute for Clinical Chemistry and Laboratory Medicine, University Regensburg, Franz-Josef-Strauss-Allee 11, 93053 Regensburg, Germany; e-mail: gerd.schmitz@klinik.uni-regensburg.de

Elisabeth Steinhagen-Thiessen, Charité, Medical Faculty of Humboldt University of Berlin, Virchow-Clinic, Medizinische Poliklinik, LDL-Apherese, Mittelallee 11, 13353 Berlin, Germany; e-mail: Elisabeth.Steinhagen-Thiessen@charite.de

Hans-Peter Thomas, Charité, Medical Faculty of Humboldt University of Berlin, Virchow-Clinic, Medizinische Poliklinik, LDL-Apherese, Mittelallee 11, 13353 Berlin, Germany; e-mail: hans-peter.thomas@charite.de

Michael Torzewski, Johannes Gutenberg-Universität Mainz, Klinikum, Institut für Klinische Chemie und Laboratoriumsmedizin, D-55101 Mainz, Germany; e-mail: torzewski@zentrallabor.klinik.uni-mainz.de

Preface

The discovery of drugs is still an unpredictable process. Breakthroughs are often the result of a combination of factors, including serendipidity, rational strategies and a few individuals with novel ideas. An encouraging development in the treatment of hypercholesterolemia has been the introduction of a new class of fungal-derived compounds that are potent competitive inhibitors of 3-hydroxy-3-methylglutaryl-coenzyme A (HMG-CoA) reductase, the rate-controlling enzyme in the biosynthetic pathway for cholesterol. HMG-CoA reductase (HMGR) inhibitors (statins) are established drugs for the treatment of hypercholesterolemia, and have been shown to induce regression of vascular atherosclerosis as well as reduction of cardiovascular-related morbidity and death in patients with and without coronary artery disease.

This book deals with statins which have substantially altered the approach to therapy of atherosclerosis and its sequelae. Emphasis is placed on the scientific background to the discoveries and the development of the therapy, with an overview of the current state of knowledge of the drugs by experts in the field. We are happy to say that invitations to these authors were gratefully accepted and each contribution constitutes an important part of this book. Each of the chapters has been designed in such a way that it can be read independently of the others, but has been written with a uniformity of theme and style that should allow smooth transitions. In the first chapter, an overview of the history and development of HMG-CoA reductase inhibitors is provided by *Stefano Bellosta*, *Rodolpho Paoletti* and *Alberto Corsini*. Although the cholesterol-lowering ability of this class of drugs is irrefutable, the mechanisms responsible for their hypocholesterolemic effects are yet to be completely defined. The goal of the following chapter written by *Margaret E. Brousseau* and *Ernst J. Schaefer* is to review the results of recent *in vitro* and *in vivo* studies that have investigated the mechanisms by which statins reduce plasma LDL concentrations, with particular emphasis on the metabolism of apoB-containing lipoproteins in humans.

Inhibition of the HMG-CoA reductase and therefore of cholesterol biosynthesis leads to an alteration of intracellular signaling cascades by modifying subcellular localisation of small G-proteins via prenylation. Other mechanisms involve the regulation of cholesterol-regulated transcription factors, as described in the third chapter (*Jörg Kotzka*, *Wilhelm Krone* and *Dirk Müller-Wieland*).

Independent of their ability to reduce plasma cholesterol, several other potential targets for statins are emerging. These targets comprise blood cells

(*Gerd Schmitz* and *Michael Torzewski*) as well as cells of the vascular wall (*Koichi Node* and *James K. Liao*). Indications and contraindications for statin treatment (primary and secondary prevention of hypercholesterolemia) are then described by *Hans-P. Thomas* and *Elisabeth Steinhagen-Thiessen*. An overview of the five large clinical trials of the beneficial effect of statins on coronary disease, which have been published since 1994, is given in the following chapter by *Helena K. Gylling* and *Tatu A. Miettinen*. The final chapter written by *Colin Berry*, *Andrew Davie* and *John McMurray* deals with the economic impact of statin therapies.

It is our hope that this book provides the reader not only with information but also stimulates further research into the pathogenesis of atherosclerosis and the mechanisms behind the action of effective statins.

Gerd Schmitz and Michael Torzewski
Regensburg, February 2002

HMG-CoA Reductase Inhibitors
ed. by G. Schmitz and M. Torzewski

History and development of HMG-CoA reductase inhibitors

Stefano Bellosta, Rodolfo Paoletti and Alberto Corsini

Department of Pharmacological Sciences, University of Milan, via Balzaretti 9, 20133 Milan, Italy

Introduction

Coronary heart disease (CHD) is the leading cause of mortality in Western countries [1, 2]. A strong, positive correlation between high levels of plasma total and low-density lipoprotein (LDL) cholesterol and CHD is well established [3]. Dietary and/or pharmacological approaches aimed at lowering elevated plasma LDL appears therefore to be a logical intervention to reduce incidence of CHD or even reversing the development of coronary atherosclerosis [1, 4–8]. A number of cholesterol-lowering drugs are currently available for human use [1, 2, 9]. Among these, 3-hydroxy-3-methylglutaryl coenzyme A (HMG-CoA) reductase inhibitors, the so-called statins: atorvastatin, cerivastatin[1], fluvastatin, pitavastatin, pravastatin, lovastatin, rosuvastatin and simvastatin, can achieve relatively large reductions in plasma cholesterol levels and are a well-established class of drugs for the treatment of hypercholesterolemia [10]. Clinical trials have demonstrated that they can induce regression of vascular atherosclerosis, as well as reduction of cardiovascular-related morbidity and mortality, in patients with and without coronary artery disease CAD [11–21]. These trials provide a powerful endorsement of the value of lipid-lowering therapy with a statin in patients who are at risk for CAD.

The beneficial effects of HMG-CoA reductase (HMGR) inhibitors are usually assumed to result from their ability to reduce cholesterol synthesis [22]. However, since mevalonic acid, the product of the effect of HMGR on HMG-CoA, is the precursor not only of cholesterol but also of numerous metabolites (Fig. 1) [23, 24], inhibition of HMGR has the potential to result in pleiotropic effects [25–28]. The beneficial effect of statins on clinical events may therefore involve non-lipid-related mechanisms that modify endothelial function, inflammatory responses, plaque stability and thrombus formation [25–30].

The purpose of this review is to summarize and discuss the steps that led to the discovery and development of the inhibitors of HMGR.

---

[1] In August 2001, Cerivastatin has been withdrawn from worldwide sale in the light of drug-interactions concern.

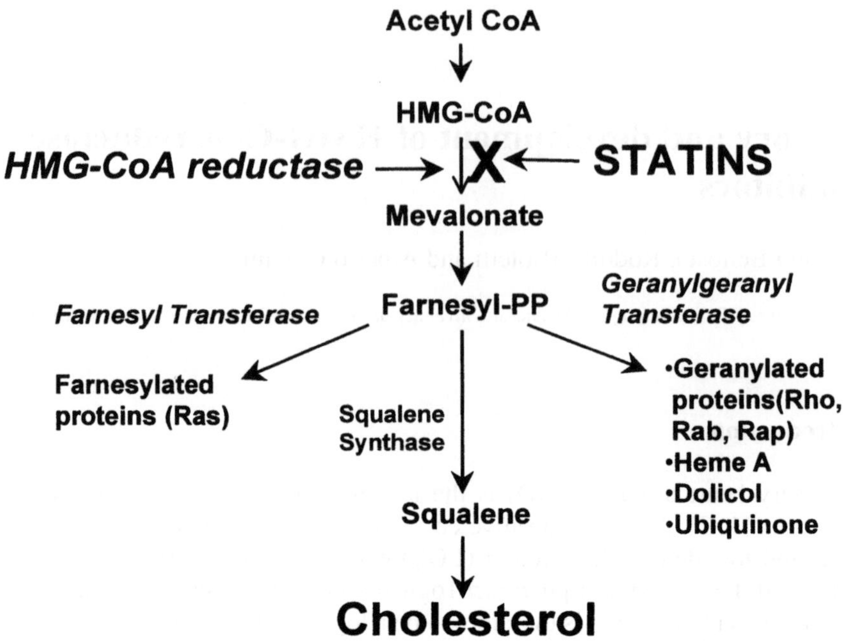

Figure 1. The mammalian cell mevalonate pathway. Legend: CoA, coenzyme A; HMG-CoA, 3-hydroxy-3-methylglutaryl coenzyme A; PP, pyrophosphate.

History and discovery of HMG-CoA reductase inhibitors

An encouraging development in the treatment of hypercholesterolemia has been the introduction of a new class of fungal-derived compounds that are potent competitive inhibitors of HMGR, the rate-controlling enzyme in the biosynthetic pathway for cholesterol (Fig. 2).

In the early '70s, Endo and Kuroda, while searching for HMGR inhibitors of microbial origin, assayed over 6,000 microbial strains for their ability to block lipid synthesis. In particular, culture broths effective in inhibiting early stages, between acetate and mevalonate, of the cholesterol synthetic pathway were further investigated in order to identify the main active component(s). In 1976 Endo and Kuroda [31] reported that citrinin, an antibiotic isolated from *Phytium ultimum,* acted as an inhibitor of cholesterol synthesis in rat liver. Further work from the same authors [32] led to the isolation of three fungal metabolites (ML-236 A, B and C) produced by *Penicillium citrinum.* ML-236B (compactin, mevastatin), was also isolated by Brown et al. from *Penicillium brevicompactum* [33].

The structure of mevastatin was determined by a combination of spectroscopic, chemical, and X-ray crystallographic methods [32]. Mevastatin has a hexahydronaphthalene skeleton substituted with a β-hydroxy-δ-lactone moi-

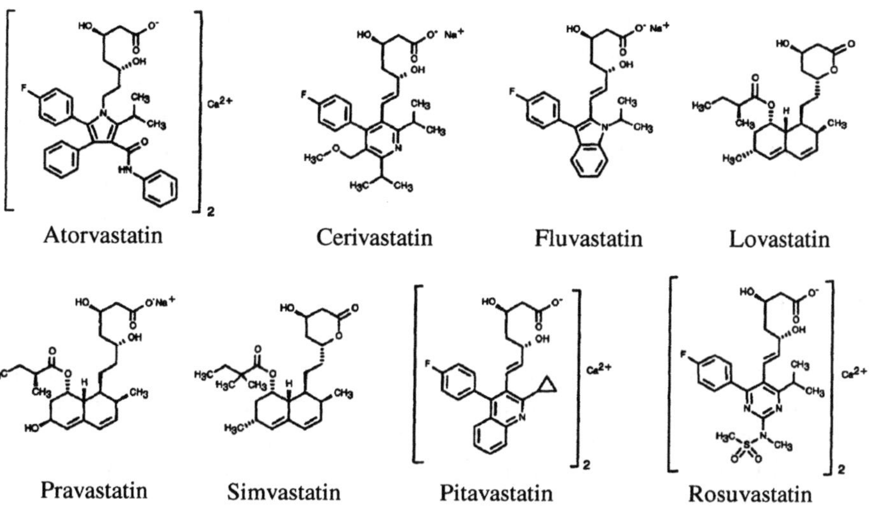

Figure 2. Chemical structure of statins.

ety, which can be converted into the water-soluble open acid by treatment with alkali [34].

ML-236 B, when administered to rats, at 5 and 20 mg kg^{-1} as a single dose, effectively reduced plasma cholesterol and [^{14}C]acetate incorporation into digitonin-precipitable sterols [32]. Endo, Kuroda and Tanzawa [34] further investigated the action of ML-236 B: this compound inhibited cholesterol synthesis from acetate, acetyl-CoA and HMG-CoA, but failed to affect the conversion of mevalonate into sterols, thus suggesting a specificity of action on HMGR. Enzyme kinetic studies showed that the compound acted as a competitive inhibitor of the HMGR due to the similarity of the open lactone acid form to 3-hydroxy-3-methylglutarate (Fig. 2). This hypothesis is further stressed by the observation that, *in vitro,* the lactone form is much less effective than the open acid form of the molecule [34].

Since this original discovery, a number of compounds that are competitive inhibitors of HMGR have appeared. In 1979 Endo isolated monacolin K (lovastatin) from a culture of *Monascus ruber* [35] and the same compound was also isolated from *Aspergillus terreus* in 1980 by Alberts and coworkers [36]. The structure of this compound differs from compactin in the presence of a methyl group at position 6 (Fig. 2).

Subsequently, the search for additional HMGR inhibitors was continued for several years, leading to the isolation of several compounds of the mevastatin family [34]. Among them, pravastatin is a ring hydroxylated metabolite of mevastatin, originally isolated from the urine of mevastatin-treated dogs. This drug is now obtained by microbial hydroxylation of mevastatin [37]. Simvastatin is synthesized directly from lovastatin by replacement of the

2-methylbutanoyl side chain with a 2,2-dimethylbutanoyl group [38]. Lovastatin and simvastatin are prodrugs that are enzymatically hydrolyzed *in vivo* to the open ring form, while pravastatin is in the active, open ring, form. Fluvastatin, which is a racemate, is the first entirely synthetic HMGR inhibitor, which differs from the original structure in its lipophilic moiety [39]. More recently, several fully HMGR synthetic enantiomeric inhibitors (Fig. 2) are being developed or are already in clinical testing.

HMG-CoA reductase

The enzyme HMGR catalyzes the NADPH-dependent reduction of HMG-CoA to mevalonate. This reaction is the committed step in cholesterol biosynthesis and is a target for intervention in the treatment of hypercholesterolemia [23].

HMG-CoA binds the reductase first to form a binary complex which in turn, upon NADPH binding, evolved into a ternary complex [40].

The overall reaction can be divided into three steps. The first reduction results in the formation of a mevaldyl-CoA hemy-thioacetal intermediate. This intermediate decomposes to mevaldehyde and $CoAS^-$ and is subsequently protonated. A second NADPH molecule then replaces $NADP^+$ and reduces mevaldehyde to mevalonate [41].

HMG-CoA reductase is a 97 kDa integral membrane protein of the endoplasmic reticulum with 8 transmembrane spans [42]. Previous studies demonstrated that the membrane-spanning regions of this enzyme are necessary for the regulated degradation of the enzyme [43–45].

Human HMGR consists of a single polypeptide chain of 888 amino acids. The aminoterminal 339 residues are membrane-bound and reside in the endoplasmic reticulum membrane projecting into the cytoplasm. The catalytic activity of the protein resides in its cytoplasmic, soluble C-terminal portion (residues 460-888). A linker region (residues 340–459) connects the two portions of the protein [46].

The crystal structure of the catalytic portion of HMGR has been determined recently with bound reaction substrates and products. The structure illustrates how HMG-CoA and NADPH are recognized and suggests a catalytic mechanism. Catalytic portions of human HMGR form tight tetramers, explaining the influence of the enzyme's oligomeric state on the activity and suggesting a mechanism for cholesterol sensing [46].

The enzyme forms tetramers with approximate D2 symmetry. The individual monomers wind around each other in an intricate fashion. The monomers are arranged in two dimers, each of which has two active sites. Residues from both monomers (called α and β) form the active sites [46]. At each active site, the HMG moiety of one HMG-CoA molecule, which is bound predominantly to a single monomer, comes into the proximity of the nicotinamide ring of an NADPH molecule, whose binding pocket is located in the neighboring monomer [41]. Thus, the active sites are positioned at the interface of the two monomers of a dimer. The formation of the tetramer does not appear to be involved in substrate binding.

HMGR is among the most highly regulated enzymes known [23]. Transcription and translation of HMGR increase when the concentrations of products of the mevalonate pathway are low. Conversely, when sterol concentrations are high, the intracellular HMGR concentration decreases rapidly [47]. A third level of regulation is achieved by phosphorylation of S872 (human enzyme) by AMP-activated protein kinase, which decreases the enzyme's activity [48]. Finally, Simoni and colleagues [49] have recently shown that HMGR is degraded in endoplasmic reticulum membranes prepared from sterol pretreated cells and that such degradation is catalyzed by a cathepsin L-type cysteine protease within the reductase membrane domain. Cathepsin L-dependent proteolysis was observed to occur preferentially in sterol-pretreated cells, suggesting that sterol treatment results in conformational changes in HMGR that make it more susceptible to such cleavage. Therefore, this enzyme is highly regulated at the level of synthesis, as well as at the level of degradation, of the protein [50, 51].

For the above-mentioned reasons HMGR appeared to be an ideal target for agents affecting cholesterol synthesis to be used in therapy.

Inhibition of HMG-CoA reductase by statins

All statins share an HMG-like moiety, which may be present in an inactive lactone form (Fig. 2). *In vivo*, these prodrugs are enzymatically hydrolyzed to their active hydroxy-acid forms [52]. The statins share rigid, hydrophobic groups that are covalently linked to the HMG-like moiety.

Relative lipophilicity estimated for the dihydroxy acid form of all statins clearly show that pravastatin and rosuvastatin are very hydrophilic as compared to other statins (Tab. 1).

In vitro *activity of HMGR inhibitors: effects on cell-free systems*

The activity of HMGR inhibitors on enzymatic activity was first shown on microsomal extracts from rat liver [34]. This study demonstrated that the inhibitory effect is competitive with respect to HMG-CoA, but is not competitive with respect to NADPH, indicating that the two substrates bind the enzyme in a coordinated fashion. The binding is reversible, therefore the drug detaches from the enzyme upon dilution. The potency of HMGR competitive inhibitors is related to a slow binding step to the enzyme [53], which triggers the formation of the final complex.

Endo et al. investigated the specificity of mevastatin using rat liver cytosol [34]. Mevastatin (5 and 50 μM), sharply reduced the incorporation of acetate, acetyl CoA and HMG-CoA into sterols by 25 and 70% respectively; meval-

Table 1. Inhibition of rat microsomal HMG-CoA reductase activity by statins and their relative lipophilicity

Inhibitor	*Ki* (M)	*ClogP*
Compactin	1.4×10^{-9}	3.85
Atorvastatin	7.5×10^{-9}	4.06
Cerivastatin	[2] 1.3×10^{-9}	1.47
Fluvastatin	0.3×10^{-9}	3.24
Lovastatin	0.6×10^{-9}	4.27
Pitavastatin	1.7×10^{-9}	1.50
Pravastatin	2.3×10^{-9}	−0.22
Rosuvastatin	12×10^{-9}	[3] −0.33
Simvastatin	0.12×10^{-9}	4.68
HMG-CoA	*Km* 1.4×10^{-6}	

[2] In the same experimental condition lovastatin has been shown to be 100-fold less potent [57].
[3] Log D [58].

onate incorporation into sterols, however, was not affected [34]. This is consistent with a specific inhibition of HMGR without any effect on later steps of cholesterol biosynthesis. Similar data have been obtained with other HMGR inhibitors [36, 39, 54–58].

The K_i (inhibition constant) values for the statin-enzyme complexes using a rat microsomal preparation range between 0.1 to 12 nM (Tab. 1) [36, 39, 52, 54–58], whereas the Michaelis constant, K_m, for HMG-CoA is 4 μM [59]. Similar potencies have been obtained using microsomal HMG-CoA reductase from hamster liver, dog liver, human hepatoma HepG2 cells and purified human catalytic domain [56–58, 60, 61].

More recently, Istvan and Deisenhofer have determined the structures of the catalytic portion of human HMGR complexed with six different statins [62]. To determine how statins prevent the binding of HMG-CoA, they solved six crystal structures of the catalytic portion of human HMGR bound to six different statin inhibitors. The structures illustrate that statins inhibit HMGR by binding to the active site of the enzyme, thus sterically preventing substrate from binding. This agrees well with kinetic studies that indicate that statins competitively inhibit HMG-CoA, but do not affect NADPH binding [34]. The study by Istvan and Deisenhofer [62] reveals also how the bulky, hydrophobic compounds of statins occupy the HMG-binding pocket and part of the binding surface for CoA. Thus, access of the substrate HMG-CoA to HMGR is blocked when statins are bound. The tight binding of statins is probably due to the large number of van der Waals interactions between inhibitors and with HMGR. The structurally diverse, rigid hydrophobic groups of the statins are accommodated in a shallow non-polar groove that is present only when COOH-residues of HMGR are disordered [62].

Effect on cultured cells

Statins effectively inhibit cholesterol synthesis in a number of cultured mammalian cells. All statins, except pravastatin and rosuvastatin, inhibit cholesterol synthesis to a similar degree *in vitro* in a number of peripheral cell lines. Much higher doses of pravastatin and rosuvastatin are required, indicating that in extra-hepatic tissues the cellular uptake of these drugs is severely impaired by their hydrophilicity. The efficacy of pravastatin and rosuvastatin in inhibiting cholesterol synthesis in human and rat hepatocytes to a degree comparable to other statins, however, suggests that specific uptake occurs in these cells. Several authors [58, 63, 64] have demonstrated the presence of a carrier that facilitates the entry of statins into hepatocytes. It is important to note that the human hepatoma HepG2 cell line does not possess a specific transporter for statins. Indeed, it has been reported that higher concentrations of hydrophilic statins, comparable to those used in peripheral cells, are required to inhibit cholesterol synthesis in HepG2 cells compared with those utilized in rat hepatocytes [56].

Surprisingly, incubation of the cells with HMGR inhibitors causes a several-fold increase of HMGR mass [65]. The competitive block of enzymatic activity, in fact, stimulates the *de novo* synthesis of HMGR, thus leading to an accumulation of the enzyme in cells [66, 67]. The build-up of HMGR in the cells is also due to a stabilization of the enzyme by statins. Edwards et al. [68] demonstrated that lovastatin increases the enzyme half-life from 2 to more than 10 h.

These results implicated a nonsterol mevalonate metabolite as having an important role in the degradation of HMGR. Studies that used either inhibitors that acted on more distal enzymatic steps in the isoprenoid/cholesterol pathway, or those in which analogs of farnesyl diphosphate were added to cells, were consistent with the proposal that the nonsterol component was derived from farnesyl diphosphate. This mechanism contributes significantly to the accumulation of the enzyme within the cell and can be regarded as an attempt by the cells to overcome the shortage of mevalonate-derived compounds that are essential for cellular homeostasis and growth [23].

In vivo activity of HMGR inhibitors

Inhibitors of cholesterol synthesis

The *in vivo* inhibition of HMGR by statins has been demonstrated in a number of animal species from mouse to monkey. The effect can be detected by determining the *in vivo* rate of incorporation of precursors into cholesterol [52].

The dose required to achieve significant reduction of cholesterol synthesis with statins is in the range of 0.01–20 mg Kg^{-1} day^{-1} both in acute and subchronic studies. Not every species, however, will respond to the administration of statins with a reduction of plasma cholesterol levels. The rat, for instance, can up-regulate cholesterol synthesis to a point at which the hypocholesterolemic effect of these drugs is overcome by the high amount of HMGR synthesized [52], thus keeping a "normal" rate of cholesterol synthesis also in the presence of competitive inhibitors [52]. On the other hand, several animal species cannot modulate their cholesterol synthesis as effectively as the rat [69]; this will result in the lowering of plasma cholesterol.

Hypolipidemic activity

Statins are effective hypocholesterolemic compounds in several animal species. The hypocholesterolemic activity has been reported in rat, hamsters, hen, rabbits, minipigs, dogs, guinea pigs, and monkeys. Doses ranging from 5 to 50 mg Kg^{-1} day^{-1} elicit reductions of plasma cholesterol from 15 to 60% [52, 70]. Among lipoprotein classes apoB- and apoE-containing lipoproteins, mainly LDL and HDL subclasses, are preferentially modulated.

The hypotriglyceridemic effect of statins can be also detected in animal species [57, 70, 71].

Pleiotropic effects of HMGR inhibitors

Clinical trials have firmly established that HMGR inhibitors can induce regression of vascular atherosclerosis, as well as reduction of cardiovascular-related morbidity and death, in patients with and without CAD. These beneficial effects on coronary events have generally been attributed to the hypocholesterolemic properties of statins. However, because mevalonate, the product of the enzyme reaction, is the precursor not only of cholesterol but also of many nonsteroidal isoprenoid compounds, inhibition of HMGR may result in pleiotropic effects [10, 23, 24, 27]. Indeed, the mevalonate pathway yields a series of isoprenoids (Fig. 1) that are vital for diverse cellular functions. These isoprenoids include: isopentenyl adenosine, present in some types of transfer RNA; dolichols, required for glycoprotein synthesis; polyisoprenoid side chains of ubiquinone and heme A, involved in electron transport [23, 24]. Several proteins post-translationally modified by the covalent attachment of mevalonate-derived isoprenoid groups, either farnesyl- or geranylgeranyl-pyrophosphate, have been identified [23, 72, 73]. These proteins must be prenylated as a prerequisite for membrane association, which is required for their function [72, 73]. Members of this family are involved in a number of cellular processes including cell signaling, cell differentiation and proliferation, myelination, cytoskeleton dynamics and endocytotic/exocytotic transport (Tab. 2). Hence, through the inhibition of HMGR, statins could affect several

Table 2. Role of prenylated proteins in cellular functioning

Molecular weight (kDa)	Comments
Farnesylated	
66–72	Nuclear laminin family
53–55	Unidentified proteins
41–46	Inositol triphosphate 5-phosphatase 2',3'-cyclic nucleotide 3'-phosphatase
37	Peroxisomal protein
21–28	Ras. Involved in cell proliferation and differentiation
Geranylgeranylated*	
21–28	Rho/Rac/Cdc42. Involved in cytoskeletal assembly, superoxide generation, cell cycle progression
	Rab. Involved in transport of vesicles
	Rap. Involved in cellular replication, platelet activation, generation of oxygen radicals
5–8	G proteins (γ-subunit). Involved in signal transduction

* In mammalian cells, 0.5–1% of total cellular proteins are geranylgeranylated.

processes that may help to explain their non-lipid-related pharmacological properties.

Atherosclerosis is a complex multifactorial process resulting from an excessive inflammatory/fibroproliferative response to various form of injurious stimuli to the arterial wall [74]. The potential interactions of cells, cytokines, and growth-regulatory molecules among the different cells in the atherosclerotic lesion present numerous opportunities for modulating lesion formation and progression [74–76].

Indeed, this possibility is supported by a variety of experimental data, indicating that statins can interfere with major events involved in the formation of atherosclerotic lesions, independently of their hypocholesterolemic properties [26, 77–80].

The beneficial effect of statins on clinical events may involve non-lipid-related mechanisms that modify endothelial function, inflammatory responses, oxidative modification of circulating lipoproteins, foam cell formation, smooth muscle cell activation, angiogenesis, plaque stability and thrombus formation [10, 28]. The pleiotropic profiles of statins are summarized in Table 3, (for an updated review of the pleiotropic effects of statins please refer to ref. [30]), and they can probably be explained by the modulation of the mevalonate pathway, because starvation of mevalonate (as a result of the inhibition of HMGR by statins) has consequences for cellular function that extend beyond decreased cholesterol synthesis. The available data demonstrate that HMGR inhibitors, beyond their lipid-lowering properties, exert a direct anti-atherosclerotic effect

Table 3. Potential mechanisms for a direct vascular action of statins

Lipid effects independent of LDL-cholesterol lowering	
	Inhibition of mevalonate biosynthesis [81]
	Increased uptake and degradation of LDL [23]
	Inhibition of LDL oxidation [82]
	Inhibition of scavenger receptor expression [83]
	Inhibition of lipoprotein secretion [84]
	Inhibition of modified LDL endocytosis [85]
Anti-atherosclerotic effects	
	Inhibition of migration and proliferation of arterial myocytes [25, 86–88]
	Inhibition of macrophage growth [89]
	Inhibition of cholesterol accumulation in macrophages [26, 85, 90]
	Inhibition of metalloproteinase secretion [25]
	Inhibition of cell adhesion [91]
	Inhibition of tissue factor expression and activity [92]
	Inhibition of superoxide generation [93]
	Decreased platelet activation [94]
	Inhibition of leukocyte-endothelium adhesion [95]
	Inhibition of chemokine and MCP-1 secretion [96–98]
	Increased fibrinolytic activity [99]
	Induction of myocyte apoptosis in proliferative lesions [100–102]
	Increased expression and activity of nitric oxide synthase [94, 124–127]
Other non lipid-related effects	
	Inhibition of CRP secretion [103]
	Inhibition of LFA-1 [104]
	Upregulation of PPARα and PPARγ [105–107]
	Increased bone formation *in vitro* and in rodents [108]
	Inhibition of intracellular Ca^{2+} mobilization [109, 110]
	Inhibition of tumor growth [111–114]
	Modulation of angiogenesis [115, 116]
	Reduction of the risk of developing dementia [117]
	Amelioration of angiotensin II-induced cardiac injury [118]

CRP, C reactive protein; LDL, low-density lipoprotein; LFA-1, leukocyte function antigen-1; MCP-1, monocyte chemotactic protein-1; PPAR, peroxisome proliferator-activated receptor.

on the arterial wall that could significantly prevent cardiovascular disease. Several issues remain to be addressed, however, before drawing any conclusion on the actual therapeutic benefit of the pleiotropic effects of statins, particularly in view of the high doses of statins required to achieve some of these effects. So far, only little evidence is available in the clinical setting (Tab. 4).

Table 4. Clinical evidence of non-lipid related effects of statins

1. Anti-inflammatory effects [95, 96, 103, 123]
2. Improvement of endothelial function [121, 122]
3. Inhibition of SMC proliferation [119, 120]

Conclusions

3-hydroxy-3-methylglutaryl coenzyme A reductase (HMGR) catalyzes the committed step in cholesterol biosynthesis, the synthesis of mevalonate from HMG-CoA. Statins are potent and effective inhibitors of HMGR, with an inhibition constant in the nanomolar range. Statins occupy a portion of the binding site of HMG-CoA, thus blocking its access to the active site of HMGR. They effectively lower serum cholesterol levels and are widely used in the treatment of hypercholesterolemia.

Although the statins that are currently available excel in reducing the biosynthesis of mevalonate, the precursor of cholesterol, it is conceivable that the recent data that gave the possibility to visualize statins bound to HMGR will facilitate the development of even better inhibitors. The beneficial effects of statins are assumed to result from their ability to reduce cholesterol biosynthesis. However, since mevalonate metabolism yields a series of isoprenoids that are vital for diverse cellular functions, ranging from cholesterol synthesis to growth control, inhibition of HMGR may result in pleiotropic effects. Indeed, the data reported by several authors show that some statins can interfere with major events involved in the formation of atherosclerotic lesions, as well as on tumor growth, independently of their hypolipidemic properties. The contribution of these direct vascular effects to the cardiovascular event reduction observed in clinical trials of statins represents one of the major challenges for future studies in order to understand the pharmacological non-lipid-related benefits of these agents.

References

1 Executive summary of the third report of the National Cholesterol Education Program (NECP) expert panel on detection, evaluation, and treatment of high blood cholesterol in adults (Adult Treatment Panel III). (2001) *JAMA* 285: 2486–2509

2 2nd Joint Task Force of European, other Societies on Coronary Prevention (1998) Prevention of coronary heart disease in clinical practice. *Eur Heart J* 19: 1434–1503

3 Brown MS, Goldstein JL (1986) A receptor-mediated pathway for cholesterol homeostasis. *Science* 232: 34–47

4 Frick MH, Elo O, Haapa K, Heinonen OP, Heinsalim P, Helo P, Huttunen JK, Kaitainemi P, Koskinen P, Maunien V et al (1987) Helsinki Heart Study: primary prevention trial with gemfibrozil in middle-aged men with dyslipidemia. *N Engl J Med* 317: 1237–1245

5 Watts GF, Lewis B, Brunt JNH, Lewis ES, Coltart DJ, Smith LDR, Mann JI, Swan AV (1992) Effects on coronary artery disease of lipid-lowering diet, or diet plus cholestyramine, in the St Thomas' Atherosclerosis Regression Study (STARS). *Lancet* 339: 563–569

6 Lipid Research Clinics Coronary Primary Prevention Trial: Results II (1984) The relationship of reduction in incidence of coronary heart disease to cholesterol lowering. *JAMA* 251: 365–374

7 Buchwald H, Varco RL, Matts JP, Long JM, Fitch LL, Campbell GS, Pearce MB, Yellin AE, Edmiston WA, Smink RD et al for the PSCH group (1990) Effect of partial ileal bypass surgery on mortality and morbidity from coronary heart disease in patients with hypercholesterolemia. *N Engl J Med* 323: 946–955

8 Kane JP, Malloy MJ, Ports TA, Phillips NR, Diehl JC, Havel RJ (1990) Regression of coronary atherosclerosis during treatment of familial hypercholesterolemia with combined drug regimens. *JAMA* 264: 3007–3012

9 Knopp RH (1999) Drug treatment of lipid disorders. *N Engl J Med* 341: 498–511
10 Corsini A, Bellosta S, Baetta R, Fumagalli R, Bernini F (1999) New insights into the pharmacodynamics and pharmacokinetic properties of statins. *Pharmacol Ther* 84: 413–428
11 Brown BG, Zhao XQ, Sacco DE, Albers JJ (1993) Lipid lowering and plaque regression: new insights into prevention of plaque disruption and clinical events in coronary disease. *Circulation* 87: 1781–1791
12 Downs JR, Clearfield M, Weis S, Whitney E, Shapiro DR, Beere PA, Langendorfer A, Stein EA, Kruyer W, Gotto AM Jr (1998) Primary prevention of acute coronary events with lovastatin in men and women with average cholesterol levels: results of AFCAPS/TexCAPS. *JAMA* 279: 1615–1622
13 Herd JA, Ballantyne CM, Farmer JA, Ferguson JJ 3rd, Jones PH, West MS, Gould KL, Gotto AM Jr (1997) Effects of fluvastatin on coronary atherosclerosis in patients with mild to moderate cholesterol elevations [Lipoprotein and Coronary Atherosclerosis Study (LCAS)]. *Am J Cardiol* 80: 278–286
14 Jukema JW, Bruschke AV, van Boven AJ, Reiber JH, Bal ET, Zwinderman AH, Jansen H, Boerma GJ, van Rappard FM, Lie KI et al (1995) Effects of lipid lowering by pravastatin on progression and regression of coronary artery disease in symptomatic men with normal to moderately elevated serum cholesterol levels: the Regression Growth Evaluation Statin Study (REGRESS). *Circulation* 91: 2528–2540
15 Long-term intervention with pravastatin in ischaemic disease (LIPID) study group (1998) Prevention of cardiovascular events and death with pravastatin in patients with coronary heart disease and a broad range of initial cholesterol levels. *N Engl J Med* 339: 1349–1357
16 Riegger G, Abletshauser C, Ludwig M, Schwandt P, Widimsky J, Weidinger G, Welzel D (1999) The effect of fluvastatin on cardiac events in patients with symptomatic coronary artery disease during one year of treatment. *Atherosclerosis* 144: 263–270
17 Sacks FM, Pfeffer MA, Moye LA, Rouleau JL, Rutherford JD, Cole TG (1996) The effect of pravastatin on coronary events after myocardial infarction in patients with average cholesterol levels. *N Engl J Med* 335: 1001–1009
18 Scandinavian Simvastatin Survival Study Group (1994) Randomised trial of cholesterol lowering in 4444 patients with coronary heart disease: the Scandinavian Simvastatin Survival Study (4S). *Lancet* 344: 1383–1389
19 Shepherd J, Cobbe SM, Ford I, Isles CG, Lorimer AR, MacFarlane PW, McKillop JH, Packard CJ (1995) Prevention of coronary heart disease with pravastatin in men with hypercholesterolemia. West of Scotland Coronary Prevention Study Group. *N Engl J Med* 333: 1301–1307
20 Pitt B, Waters D, Brown WV, van Boven AJ, Schwartz L, Title LM, Eisenberg D, Shurzinske L, McCormick LS (1999) Aggressive lipid-lowering therapy compared with angioplasty in stable coronary artery disease. Atorvastatin *versus* revascularization treatment investigators. *N Engl J Med* 341: 70–76
21 Schwartz GG, Olsson AG, Ezekowitz MD, Ganz P, Oliver MF, Waters D, Zeiher A, Chaitman BR, Leslie S, Stern T (2001) Myocardial Ischemia Reduction with Aggressive Cholesterol Lowering (MIRACL) Study Investigators Effects of atorvastatin on early recurrent ischemic events in acute coronary syndromes: the MIRACL study: a randomized controlled trial. *JAMA* 285: 1711–1718
22 Feussner G (1994) HMG-CoA reductase inhibitors. *Curr Opin Lipidol* 5: 59–68
23 Goldstein JL, Brown MS (1990) Regulation of the mevalonate pathway. *Nature* 343: 425–430
24 Grunler J, Ericsson J, Dallner G (1994) Branch-point reactions in the biosynthesis of cholesterol, dolichol, ubiquinone and prenylated proteins. *Biochim Biophys Acta* 1212: 259–277
25 Bellosta S, Bernini F, Ferri N, Quarato P, Canavesi M, Arnaboldi L, Fumagalli R, Paoletti R, Corsini A (1998) Direct vascular effects of HMG-CoA reductase inhibitors. *Atherosclerosis* 137 (Suppl): S101–S109
26 Bernini F, Didoni G, Bonfadini G, Bellosta S, Fumagalli R (1993) Requirement for mevalonate in acetylated LDL induction of cholesterol esterification in macrophages. *Atherosclerosis* 104: 19–26
27 Corsini A, Mazzotti M, Raiteri M, Soma MR, Gabbiani G, Fumagalli R, Paoletti R (1993) Relationship between mevalonate pathway and arterial myocyte proliferation: *in vitro* studies with inhibitors of HMG-CoA reductase. *Atherosclerosis* 101: 117–125
28 Rosenson RS, Tangney C (1998) Antiatherothrombotic properties of statins. *JAMA* 279: 1643–1650
29 Bellosta S, Ferri N, Bernini F, Paoletti R, Corsini A (2000) Non-lipid-related effects of statins. *Ann Med* 32: 164–176

30 Comparato C, Altana C, Bellosta S, Baetta R, Paoletti R, Corsini A (2001) Clinically relevant pleiotropic effects of statins: drug properties or effect of profound cholesterol reduction? *Nutr Metab Cardiovasc Dis* 11: 328–343
31 Endo A, Kuroda M (1976) Citrinin, an inhibitor of cholesterol synthesis. *J Antibiot* 29: 841–843
32 Endo A, Kuroda M, Tsujita Y (1976) ML-236A, ML-236B and ML-236C, new inhibitors of cholesterogenesis produced by *Penicillium citrinum*. *J Antibiot* 29: 1346–1348
33 Brown AG, Smale TC, King TJ, Hasenkamp R, Thompson RH (1976) Crystal and molecular structure of compactin, a new antifungal metabolite from *Penicillium brevicompactum*. *J Chem Soc Perkin* I: 1165–1170
34 Endo A, Kuroda M, Tanzawa K (1976) Competitive inhibition of 3-hydroxy-3-methylglutaryl coenzyme A reductase by ML-236A and ML-236B, fungal metabolites, having hypocholesterolemic activity. *FEBS Lett* 72: 323–326
35 Endo A (1979) Monacolin K, a new hypocholesterolemic agent produced by *Monascus* species. *J Antibiot* 32: 852–854
36 Alberts AW, Chen J, Kuron G, Hunt V, Huff J, Hoffmann C, Rothrock J, Lopez M, Joshua H, Harris E et al (1980) Mevinolin: a highly potent competitive inhibitor of hydroxy-methylglutaryl-coenzyme A reductase and a cholesterol-lowering agent. *Proc Natl Acad Sci USA* 77: 3957–3961
37 Arai M, Serizawa N, Terhara A, Tsujita Y, Tanaka M, Masuda H, Ishikawa S (1988) Pravastatin sodium (CS-514), a novel cholesterol lowering agent which inhibits HMG-CoA reductase. *Sankyo Kenkyusho Nempo* 40: 1–38
38 Hoffmann WF, Alberts AW, Cragoe EJ, Deanna AA, Evans BE, Gilfillan JL, Gould NP, Huff JW, Novello FC, Prugh JD et al (1986) 3-hydroxy-3-methylglutaryl Coenzyme A reductase inhibitors. 2. Structural modifications of 7-(substituted aryl)-3,5-dihydroxy-6-heptenoic acids and their lactone derivatives. *J Med Chem* 29: 159–169
39 Kathawala FG (1991) HMG-CoA reductase inhibitors: an exciting development in the treatment of hyperlipoproteinemia. *Med Res Rev* 11: 121–146
40 Endo A, Tsujita Y, Kuroda M, Tanzawa K (1977) Inhibition of cholesterol synthesis *in vitro* and *in vivo* by ML-236A and ML-236B, competitive inhibitors of 3-hydroxy-3-methylglutaryl Coenzyme A reductase. *Eur J Biochem* 77: 31–36
41 Istvan ES, Palnitkar M, Buchanan SK, Deisenhofer J (2000) Crystal structure of the catalytic portion of human HMG-CoA reductase: insights into regulation of activity and catalysis. *EMBO J* 19: 819–830
42 Olender EH, Simoni RD (1992) The intracellular targeting and membrane topology of 3-hydroxy-3-methylglutaryl-CoA reductase. *J Biol Chem* 267: 4223–4235
43 Gil G, Faust JR, Chin DJ, Goldstein JL, Brown MS (1985) Membrane-bound domain of HMG CoA reductase is required for sterol-enhanced degradation of the enzyme. *Cell* 41: 249–258
44 Chun KT, Simoni RD (1992) The role of the membrane domain in the regulated degradation of 3-hydroxy-3-methylglutaryl coenzyme A reductase. *J Biol Chem* 267: 4236–4246
45 Kumagai H, Chun KT, Simoni RD (1995) Molecular dissection of the role of the membrane domain in the regulated degradation of 3-hydroxy-3-methylglutaryl coenzyme A reductase. *J Biol Chem* 270: 19,107–19,113
46 Istvan ES, Deisenhofer J (2000) The structure of the catalytic portion of human HMG-CoA reductase. *Biochim Biophys Acta* 1529: 9–18
47 Nakanishi M, Goldstein JL, Brown MS (1988) Multivalent control of 3-hydroxy-3-methylglutaryl coenzyme A reductase. Mevalonate-derived product inhibits translation of mRNA and accelerates degradation of enzyme. *J Biol Chem* 263: 8929–8937
48 Omkumar RV, Rodwell VW (1994) Phosphorylation of Ser871 impairs the function of His865 of Syrian hamster 3-hydroxy-3-methylglutaryl coenzyme A reductase. *J Biol Chem* 268: 16,862–16,866
49 Moriyama T, Wada M, Urade R, Kito M, Katunuma N, Ogawa T, Simoni RD (2001) 3-hydroxy-3 methylglutaryl coenzyme A reductase is sterol-dependently cleaved by cathepsin L-type cysteine protease in the isolated endoplasmic reticulum. *Arch Biochem Biophys* 386: 205–212
50 Moriyama T, Sather SK, McGee TP, Simoni RD (1998) Degradation of HMG-CoA reductase *in vitro*. Cleavage in the membrane domain by a membrane-bound cysteine protease. *J Biol Chem* 273: 22037–22043
51 Edwards P, Ericsson J (1999) Sterols and isoprenoids: signaling molecules derived from the cholesterol biosynthetic pathway. *Annu Rev Biochem* 68: 157–183
52 Corsini A, Maggi FM, Catapano AL (1995) Pharmacology of competitive inhibitors of HMG-CoA

reductase. *Pharmacol Res* 31: 9–27
53 Flamberg PL, Peishoff CE, Bryan DL, Leber J, Elliott JD, Metcalf BW, Mayer RJ (1990) Slow binding inhibition of 3-hydroxy-3-methylglutaryl Coenzyme A reductase. *Biochemistry* 29: 4115–4120
54 Tsujita Y, Kuroda M, Shimada Y, Tanzawa M, Kaneko I, Tanaka M, Masuda H, Turami C, Watanabe Y, Fujii S (1986) CS-514, a competitive inhibitor of 3-hydroxy-3-methylglutaryl Coenzyme A reductase: tissue-selective inhibitor of sterol synthesis and hypolipidemic effect on various animal species. *Biochim Biophys Acta* 877: 50–60
55 Aoki T, Nishimura H, Nakagawa S, Kojima J, Suzuki H, Tamaki T, Wada Y, Yokoo N, Sato F, Kimata H et al (1997) Pharmacological profile of a novel synthetic inhibitor of 3-hydroxy-3-methylglutaryl-coenzyme A reductase. *Arzneim-Forsch/Drug Res* 47 (II): 904–909
56 Shaw MK, Newton RS, Sliskovic DR, Roth B, Ferguson E, Krause BR (1990) Hep-G2 cells and primary rat hepatocytes differ in their response to inhibitors of HMG-CoA reductase. *Biochim Biophys Res Comm* 170: 726–734
57 Bischoff H, Angerbauer R, Bender J, Bischoff E, Faggiotto A, Petzinna D, Pfitzner J, Porter MC, Schmidt D, Thomas G (1997) Cerivastatin: pharmacology of a novel synthetic and highly active HMG-CoA reductase inhibitor. *Atherosclerosis* 135: 119–130
58 McTaggart F, Buckett L, Davidson R, Holdgate G, McCormick A, Schneck D, Smith G, Warwick M (2001) Preclinical and clinical pharmacology of rosuvastatin, a new 3-hydroxy-3-methylglutaryl-coenzyme A reductase inhibitor. *Am J Cardiol* 87(suppl): 28B–32B
59 Bischoff KM, Rodwell VW (1992) Biosynthesis and characterization of (S)-and (R)-3-hydroxy-3-methylglutaryl coenzyme A. *Biochem Med Metab Biol* 48: 149–158
60 Bosisio E, Cighetti G, Di Padova C, Rovagnati P, Galli Kienle M, Galli G, Paoletti R (1982) Effects of compactin (ML-236B) on biliary lipid composition and cholesterol catabolism in the hamster. *Pharmacol Res Commun* 14: 577–592
61 Alberts AW (1988) HMG-CoA reductase inhibitors. The development. *Ather Rev* 18: 123–131
62 Istvan ES, Deisenhofer J (2001) Structural mechanism for statin inhibition of HMG-CoA reductase. *Science* 292: 1160–1164
63 Komai T, Shigehara E, Tokui T, Koga T, Ishigami M, Kuroiwa C, Horiichi S (1992) Carrier-mediated uptake of pravastatin by rat hepatocytes in primary culture. *Biochem Pharmacol* 43: 667–670
64 Nakai D, Nakagomi R, Furuta Y, Tokui T, Abe T, Ikeda T, Nishimura K (2001) Human liver-specific organic anion transporter, LST-1, mediates uptake of pravastatin by human hepatocytes. *J Pharmacol Exp Ther* 297: 861–867
65 Brown MS, Faust JR, Goldstein JL, Kaneko I, Endo A (1978) Induction of 3-hydroxy-3-methylglutaryl Coenzyme A reductase activity in human fibroblasts incubated with compactin (ML-236B), a competitive inhibitor of the reductase. *J Biol Chem* 253: 1121–1128
66 Chin DJ, Luskey KL, Anderson RGW, Faust JR, Goldstein JL, Brown MS (1982) Appearance of crystalloid endoplasmic reticulum in compactin resistant Chinese hamster cells with a 500-fold increase in 3-hydroxy-3-methylglutaryl Coenzyme A reductase. *Proc Natl Acad Sci USA* 79: 1185–1189
67 Liscum L, Luskey KL, Chin DJ, Ho YK, Goldstein JL, Brown MS (1983) Regulation of 3-hydroxy-3-methylglutaryl Coenzyme A reductase and its mRNA in rat liver as studied with a monoclonal antibody and a cDNA probe. *J Biol Chem* 258: 8450–8455
68 Edwards PA, Lan SF, Fogelman AM (1983) Alteration in the rates of synthesis and degradation of rat liver 3-hydroxy-3-methylglutaryl Coenzyme A reductase produced by cholestyramine and mevinolin. *J Biol Chem* 258: 10219–10222
69 Todd PA, Goa KL (1990) Simvastatin. *Drugs* 40: 583–607
70 Suzuki H, Yamazaki H, Aoki T, Tamaki T, Sato F, Kitahara M, Saito Y (2001) Hypolipidemic effect of NK-104 and other 3-hydroxy-3-methylglutaryl coenzyme A reductase inhibitors in guinea pigs. *Arzneim-Forsch/Drug Res* 51: 38–45
71 Suzuki H, Yamazaki H, Aoki T, Kojima J, Tamaki T, Sato F, Kitahara M, Saito Y (2000) Lipid-lowering and antiatherosclerotic effect of NK-104, a potent 3-hydroxy-3-methylglutaryl coenzyme A reductase inhibitor, in Watanabe heritable hyperlipidemic rabbits. *Arzneim-Forsch/Drug Res* 50: 995–1003
72 Glomset JA, Gelb MH, Farnsworth CC (1990) Prenyl proteins in eukaryotic cells: a new type of membrane anchor. *Trends Biochem Sci* 15: 139–142
73 Maltese WA (1990) Post-translational modification of proteins by isoprenoids in mammalian cells. *FASEB J* 4: 3319–3328

74 Ross R (1999) Atherosclerosis – an inflammatory disease. *N Engl J Med* 340: 115–126
75 Wissler RW (1991) Update on the pathogenesis of atherosclerosis. *Am J Med* 91 (Suppl 1B): 1B–3S_1B–9S
76 Ip JH, Fuster V, Badimon L, Badimon J, Taubman MB, Chesebro JH (1990) Syndromes of accelerated atherosclerosis: role of vascular injury and smooth muscle cell proliferation. *J Am Coll Cardiol* 15: 1667–1687
77 Richardson PD, Davies MJ, Born GVR (1989) Influence of plaque configuration and stress distribution on fissuring of coronary atherosclerotic plaques. *Lancet* 2: 941–944
78 Burleigh MC, Briggs AD, Lendon CL, Davies MJ, Born GV, Richardson PD (1992) Collagen types I and II, collagen content, GAGs and mechanical strength of human atherosclerotic plaque caps: snap-wise variations. *Atherosclerosis* 96: 71–81
79 Dollery CM, McEwan JR, Henney AM (1995) Matrix metalloproteinases and cardiovascular disease. *Circ Res* 77: 863–868
80 Bellosta S, Via D, Canavesi M, Pfister P, Fumagalli R, Paoletti R, Bernini F (1998) HMG-CoA reductase inhibitors reduce MMP-9 secretion by macrophages. *Arterioscl Thromb Vasc Biol* 18: 1671–1678
81 Endo A (1992) The discovery and development of HMG-CoA reductase inhibitors. *J Lipid Res* 33: 1569–1582
82 Aviram M, Dankner G, Cogan U, Hochgraf E, Brook JG (1992) Lovastatin inhibits low-density lipoprotein oxidation and alters its fluidity and uptake by macrophages: *in vitro* and *in vivo* studies. *Metabolism* 41: 229–235
83 Umetani N, Kanayama Y, Okamura M, Negoro N, Takeda T (1996) Lovastatin inhibits gene expression of type-I scavenger receptor in THP-1 human macrophages. *Biochim Biophys Acta* 1303: 199–206
84 La Ville A, Moshy R, Turner PR, Miller NE, Lewis B (1984) Inhibition of cholesterol synthesis reduces low-density-lipoprotein apoprotein B production without decreasing very-low-density-lipoprotein apoprotein B synthesis in rabbits. *Biochem J* 218: 321–323
85 Bernini F, Scurati N, Bonfadini G, Fumagalli R (1995) HMG-CoA reductase inhibitors reduce acetyl LDL endocytosis in mouse peritoneal macrophages. *Arterioscl Thromb Vasc Biol* 15: 1352–1358
86 Corsini A, Arnaboldi L, Raiteri M, Quarato P, Faggiotto A, Paoletti R, Fumagalli R (1996) Effect of the new HMG-CoA reductase inhibitor cerivastatin (BAY W 6228) on migration, proliferation and cholesterol synthesis in arterial myocytes. *Pharmacol Res* 33: 56–62
87 Soma MR, Donetti E, Parolini C, Mazzini G, Ferrari C, Fumagalli R, Paoletti R (1993) HMG-CoA reductase inhibitors: *in vivo* effects on carotid intimal thickening in normocholesterolemic rabbits. *Arterioscl Thromb Vasc Biol* 13: 571–578
88 Corsini A, Bernini F, Quarato P, Donetti E, Bellosta S, Fumagalli R, Paoletti R, Soma MR (1996) Non-lipid-related effects of 3-hydroxy-3-methylglutaryl coenzyme A reductase inhibitors. *Cardiology* 87: 458–468
89 Sakai M, Kobori S, Matsumura T, Biwa T, Sato Y, Takemura T, Hakamata H, Horiuchi S, Shichiri M (1997) HMG-CoA reductase inhibitors suppress macrophage growth induced by oxidized low density lipoprotein. *Atherosclerosis* 133: 51–59
90 Cignarella A, Brennhausen B, von Eckardstein A, Assmann G, Cullen P (1998) Differential effects of lovastatin on the trafficking of endogenous and lipoprotein-derived cholesterol in human monocyte-derived macrophages. *Arterioscl Thromb Vasc Biol* 18: 1322–1329
91 Masaaki K, Kurose I, Russell J, Granger DN (1997) Effect of fluvastatin on leukocyte-endothelial cell adhesion in hypercholesterolemic rats. *Arterioscl Thromb Vasc Biol* 17: 1521–1526
92 Colli S, Eligini S, Lalli M, Camera M, Paoletti R, Tremoli E (1997) Vastatins inhibit tissue factor in cultured human macrophages: a novel mechanism of protection against atherosclerosis. *Arterioscler Thromb Vasc Biol* 17: 265–272
93 Giroux LM, Davignon J, Naruszewicz (1993) Simvastatin inhibits the oxidation of low-density lipoproteins by activated human monocyte-derived macrophages. *Biochim Biophys Acta* 1165: 335–338
94 Laufs U, Gertz K, Huang P, Nickenig G, Bohm M, Dirnagl U, Endres M (2000) Atorvastatin upregulates type III nitric oxide synthase in thrombocytes, decreases platelet activation, and protects from cerebral ischemia in normocholesterolemic mice. *Stroke* 31: 2442–2449
95 Kimura M, Kurose I, Russell J, Granger DN (1997) Effects of fluvastatin on leukocyte-endothelial cell adhesion in hypercholesterolemic rats. *Arterioscler Thromb Vasc Biol* 17: 1521–1526

96 Romano M, Diomede L, Sironi M, Massimiliano l, Sottocorno M, Polentarutti N, Guglielmotti A, Albani D, Bruno A, Fruscella P et al (2000) Inhibition of monocyte chemotactic protein-1 synthesis by statins. *Lab Invest* 80: 1095–1100
97 Ikeda U, Shimada K (1999) Statins and monocytes. *Lancet* 353: 2070
98 Terkeltaub R, Solan J, Barry MJ, Santoro D, Bokoch GM (1994) Role of the mevalonate pathway of isoprenoid synthesis in IL-8 generation by activated monocytic cells. *J Leukocyte Biol* 55: 749–755
99 Essig M, Vrtovsnik F, Nguyen G, Sraer JD, Friedlander G (1998) Lovastatin modulates *in vivo* and *in vitro* the plasminogen activator/plasmin system of rat proximal tubular cells: role of geranylgeranylation and Rho proteins. *J Am Soc Nephrol* 9: 1377–1388
100 Baetta R, Paoletti R, Fumagalli R, Soma MR (1997) Mevalonate modulation of cell proliferation and apoptosis. *Oncol Rep* 4: 257–261
101 Guijarro C, Blanco-Colio LM, Ortego M, Alonso C, Ortiz A, Plaza JJ, Diaz C, Hernandez G, Egido J (1998) 3-hydroxy-3-methylglutaryl coenzyme A reductase and isoprenylation inhibitors induce apoptosis of vascular smooth muscle cells in culture. *Circ Res* 83: 490–500
102 Baetta R, Donetti E, Comparato C, Calore M, Rossi A, Teruzzi C, Paoletti R, Fumagalli R, Soma MR (1997) Proapoptotic effect of atorvastatin on stimulated rabbit smooth muscle cells. *Pharmacol Res* 36: 115–121
103 Ridker PM, Rifai N, Pfeffer MA, Sacks F, Braunwald E (1999) Long-term effects of pravastatin on plasma concentration of C-reactive protein. *Circulation* 100: 230–235
104 Weitz-Schmidt G, Welzenbach K, Brinkmann V, Kamata T, Kallen J, Bruns C, Cottens S, Takada Y, Hommel U (2001) Statins selectively inhibit leukocyte function antigen-1 by binding to a novel regulatory integrin site. *Nat Med* 7: 687–692
105 Inoue I, Goto S, Mizotani K, Awata T, Mastunaga T, Kawai S, Nakajima T, Hokari S, Komoda T, Katayama S (2000) Lipophilic HMG-CoA reductase inhibitor has an anti-inflammatory effect: reduction of mRNA levels for interleukin-1beta, interleukin-6, cyclooxygenase-2, and p22phox by regulation of peroxisome proliferator-activated receptor alpha (PPARalpha) in primary endothelial cells. *Life Sci* 67: 863–876
106 Li AC, Brown KK, Silvestre MJ, Willson TM, Palinski W, Glass CK (2000) Peroxisome proliferator-activated receptor gamma ligands inhibit development of atherosclerosis in LDL receptor-deficient mice. *J Clin Invest* 106: 523–531
107 Fajas L, Schoonjans K, Gelman L, Kim JB, Najib J, Martin G, Fruchart JC, Briggs M, Spiegelman BM, Auwerx J (1999) Regulation of peroxisome proliferator-activated receptor gamma expression by adipocyte differentiation and determination factor 1/sterol regulatory element binding protein 1: implications for adipocyte differentiation and metabolism. *Mol Cell Biol* 19: 5495–5503
108 Mundy G, Garrett R, Harris S, Chan J, Chen D, Rossini G, Boyce B, Zhao M, Gutierrez G (1999) Stimulation of bone formation *in vitro* and in rodents by statins. *Science* 286: 1946–1949
109 Escobales N, Castro M, Altieri PI, Sanabria P (1996) Simvastatin releases Ca^{2+} from a thapsigargin-sensitive pool and inhibits InsP3-dependent Ca^{2+} mobilization in vascular smooth muscle cells. *J Cardiovasc Pharmacol* 27: 383–391
110 Yada T, Nakata M, Shiraishi T, Kakei M (1999) Inhibition by simvastatin, but not pravastatin, of glucose-induced cytosolic Ca^{2+} signaling and insulin secretion due to blockade of L-type Ca^{2+} channels in rat islet beta-cells. *Br J Pharmacol* 126: 1205–1213
111 Dunnington DJ, Prichett W, Greig R (1989) Stimulation of anchorage independent proliferation of human adrenocortical carcinoma cells by inhibition of cholesterol biosynthesis. *Biochem Biophys Res Commun* 165: 219–225
112 Perez-Sala D, Mollinedo F (1994) Inhibition of isoprenoid biosynthesis induces apoptosis in human promyelocytic HL-60 cells. *Biochem Biophys Res Commun* 199: 1209–1215
113 Guijarro C, Blanco-Colio LM, Ortego M, Alonso C, Ortiz A, Plaza JJ, Diaz C, Hernandez G, Edigo J (1998) 3-Hydroxy-3-methylglutaryl coenzyme a reductase and isoprenylation inhibitors induce apoptosis of vascular smooth muscle cells in culture. *Circ Res* 83: 490–500
114 Soma MR, Pagliarini P, Butti G, Paoletti R, Paoletti P, Fumagalli R (1992) Simvastatin, an inhibitor of cholesterol biosynthesis, shows a synergistic effect with N,N'-bis(2-chloroethyl)-N-nitrosourea and beta-interferon on human glioma cells. *Cancer Res* 52: 4348–4355
115 Vincent L, Chen W, Hong L, Mirshahi F, Mishal Z, Mirshahi-Khorassani T, Vannier J, Soria J, Soria C (2001) Inhibition of endothelial cell migration by cerivastatin, an HMG-CoA reductase inhibitor: contribution to its anti-angiogenic effect. *FEBS Lett* 495: 159–166

116 Kureishi Y, Luo Z, Shiojima I, Bialik A, Fulton D, Lefer DJ, Sessa WC, Walsh K (2000) The HMG-CoA reductase inhibitor simvastatin activities the protein kinases Akt and promotes angiogenesis in normocholesterolemic animals. *Nat Med* 6: 1004–1010
117 Jick H, Zornberg GL, Jick SS, Seshadri S, Drachman DA (2000) Statins and the risk of dementia. *Lancet* 1627–1631
118 Dechend R, Fiebeler A, Park JK, Muller DN, Theuer J, Mervaala E, Bieringer M, Gulba D, Dietz R, Luft FC et al (2001) Amelioration of angiotensin II-induced cardiac injury by a 3-hydroxy-3-methylglutaryl coenzyme A reductase inhibitor. *Circulation* 104: 576–581
119 Walter DH, Schachinger V, Elsner M, Mach S, Auch-Schwelk W, Zeiher AM (2000) Effect of statin therapy on restenosis after coronary stent implantation. *Am J Cardiol* 85: 962–968
120 Corsini A, Pazzucconi F, Pfister P, Paoletti R, Sirtori CR (1996) Inhibition of proliferation of arterial smooth-muscle cells by fluvastatin [letter]. *Lancet* 348: 1584
121 O'Driscoll G, Green D, Taylor RR (1997) Simvastatin, an HMG-coenzyme A reductase inhibitor, improves endothelial function within 1 month. *Circulation* 95: 1126–1131
122 Sheng-Fang S, Ca-Ling H, Ca-Wei C, Bai-Ching L, Tsung-Ming L (2000) Effects of pravastatin on left ventricular mass in patients with hyperlipidemia and essential hypertension. *Am J Cardiol* 86: 514–518
123 Sparrow CP, Burton CA, Hernandez M, Mundt S, Hassing H, Patel S, Rosa R, Hermanowski-Vosatka A, Wang P, Zhang D et al (2001) Simvastatin has anti-inflammatory and antiatherosclerotic activities independent of plasma cholesterol lowering. *Arterioscler Thromb Vasc Biol* 21: 115–121
124 Ni W, Egashira K, Kataoka C, Kitamoto S, Koyanagi M, Inoue S, Takeshita A (2001) Antiinflammatory and antiatherosclerotic actions of HMG-CoA reductase inhibitors in a rat model of chronic inhibition of nitric oxide synthesis. *Circ Res* 89: 415–421
125 Laufs U, La Fata V, Plutzky J, Liao JK (1998) Upregulation of endothelial nitric oxide synthase by HMG-CoA reductase inhibitors. *Circulation* 97: 1129–1135
126 Laufs U, La Fata V, Liao JK (1997) Inhibition of 3-hydroxy-3-methylglutaryl (HMG)-CoA reductase blocks hypoxia-mediated down-regulation of endothelial nitric oxide synthase. *J Biol Chem* 272: 31,725–31,729
127 Kaesemeyer WH (1999) Pravastatin sodium activates endothelial nitric oxide synthase independently of its cholesterol-lowering actions. *J Am Coll Cardiol* 33: 234–241

Structure and mechanisms of action of HMG-CoA reductase inhibitors

Margaret E. Brousseau and Ernst J. Schaefer

Lipid Metabolism Laboratory, Jean Mayer-USDA Human Nutrition Research Center on Aging, Tufts University, and Lipid Research Laboratory, Division of Endocrinology, Metabolism, Diabetes and Molecular Medicine, New England Medical Center, Boston, MA 02111, USA

Introduction

An elevated low density lipoprotein (LDL) cholesterol concentration is a major risk factor for the development of coronary heart disease (CHD) [1], which remains the leading cause of death in our society [2]. The efficacy of LDL reduction in the prevention of CHD has clearly been demonstrated in a number of primary and secondary intervention trials (reviewed in reference [3]). Inhibitors of 3-hydroxy-3-methylglutaryl coenzyme A (HMG-CoA) reductase, the rate-limiting enzyme in cholesterol biosynthesis, constitute the most powerful class of hypolipidemic drugs currently available. Treatment with HMG-CoA reductase inhibitors, or statins, has been shown to reduce plasma LDL cholesterol, apolipoprotein (apo) B, and triglyceride concentrations in a variety of hypercholesterolemic subjects [3, 4–10], while modestly increasing levels of high density lipoprotein (HDL) cholesterol [3].

Although it is irrefutable that statins significantly reduce plasma cholesterol concentrations, the mechanisms responsible for the hypocholesterolemic effects of this class of drugs are yet to be fully elucidated. On the cellular level, the inhibition of HMG-CoA reductase activity by statins has been shown to reduce hepatocyte cholesterol concentration [11] which, in turn, leads to upregulation of LDL receptor expression and, ultimately, to increased clearance of LDL and its precursors from the circulation [12, 13]. However, increased plasma clearance of LDL has not been demonstrated consistently in subjects treated with statins [7, 8, 10, 14–19], suggesting that the LDL-lowering effect of statins may also be attributable to decreased production of LDL apoB-100. This concept is further supported by the fact that statins are capable of reducing LDL levels in patients with homozygous familial hypercholesterolemia (FH), who lack functional LDL receptors [20, 21]. The goal of this work is to review the results of recent *in vitro* and *in vivo* studies that have investigated the mechanisms by which statins reduce plasma LDL concentrations, with particular emphasis on the metabolism of apoB-containing lipoproteins in humans.

Structure and pharmacology

In 1971, Akira Endo and colleagues, inspired by Alexander Fleming's discovery of the antibiotic penicillin from a mold belonging to the genus *Penicillium* some 43 years earlier, embarked on their efforts to identify a microbial product capable of inhibiting the rate-limiting step in cholesterol biosynthesis [22]. Over a 2-year period, these researchers screened 6,000 microbial strains for their ability to block lipid synthesis. Their efforts led to the discovery that a strain of *Penicillium citrinum* produced active compounds that inhibited the action of HMG-CoA reductase and, ultimately, to the identification of the first statin, mevastatin [23–25].

Since the discovery of mevastatin, additional statins have been produced by fungal fermentation (lovastatin, pravastatin, and simvastatin), while several others have been chemically synthesized (fluvastatin, atorvastatin, cerivastatin, crilvastatin, and nisvastatin). The statins share a number of common structural features: 1) each is comprised of the substrate analog in either the open-chain (pravastatin and atorvastatin) or closed-ring lactone (lovastatin, simvastatin, fluvastatin, and cerivastatin) form; 2) each has a complex hydrophobic ring structure which allows for tight binding to the reductase enzyme; and 3) each has a side group on the ring which defines its solubility and, ultimately, its pharmacokinetic properties [26]. The three statins produced by fungal fermentation share a great deal of structural homology, whereas the structures of the synthetic statins are markedly different. Not surprisingly, this structural variation contributes to the functional variation observed among the statins, as shown by the differing doses needed to achieve similar hypocholesterolemic effects. The plasma half-life of a statin also contributes to its cholesterol-reducing ability. The majority of statins have a short half-life in the plasma, ranging between 2–3 h. Two notable exclusions from this list are atorvastatin, which has the longest half-life at 14 h, and fluvastatin, which has the shortest half-life at 42 min [26]. The prolonged half-life of atorvastatin has been implicated as the source of its greater efficacy in cholesterol-lowering.

As stated above, the structure of a statin influences its solubility which, in turn, influences its distribution and uptake by cells other than those of the liver. For example, atorvastatin, lovastatin, and simvastatin are lipophilic in nature and, thus, are capable of crossing the blood-brain barrier and inducing central nervous system (CNS) disturbances, whereas cerivastatin, fluvastatin, and pravastatin are hydrophilic compounds incapable of affecting the CNS. Moreover, the lipophilic statins must first be oxidized or conjugated with polar groups to increase their solubility, prior to excretion from the body. Most statins undergo a cytochrome P450-mediated reaction in the liver. The 3A4 isoenzyme of cytochrome P450 metabolizes many of these drugs, with the exception of fluvastatin, which uses the 2C9 isoenzyme, and pravastatin which is not metabolized via the cytochrome P450 pathway [27, 28]. Cerivastatin is capable of interacting with both the 3A4 and 2C8 isoenzymes [29]. It is important to note that a variety of naturally occurring compounds, as well as pharmaceutical agents, can act as competitive substrates or inhibitors of cytochrome P450 isoenzymes [26, 30]; thus, potential interactions should be considered prior to statin administration.

Mechanisms of lipid lowering

In vitro *studies*

Several studies have been performed to investigate the effect of HMG-CoA reductase inhibitors on apoB secretion *in vitro*, the most recent of which are summarized in Table 1. In 1991, Ribeiro et al. reported the results of their experiments designed to examine the effect of simvastatin on apoB secretion, using primary cultures of rat hepatocytes [31]. When added to the culture medium at a dose of 0.10 μM for a period of 24 h, simvastatin significantly inhibited the incorporation of acetate into cholesterol and cholesteryl esters (CE), without affecting the synthesis and secretion of triglycerides. Surprisingly, simvastatin was found to stimulate both apoB synthesis and secretion. Because apoB mRNA abundance was not simultaneously increased in the statin-treated hepatocytes, it can be inferred that the simvastatin-induced changes in apoB synthesis occurred at the post-transcriptional level.

In experiments similar to those of Ribeiro et al. [31], Qin and colleagues assessed the effects of simvastatin (0.01 to 1.5 μM) on cholesterolgenesis and apoB secretion in primary cultures of rat and human hepatocytes, as well as in HepG2 cells [32]. Incubation of rat hepatocytes with 0.1 μM of simvastatin was shown to inhibit cholesterol synthesis by 73%, with a dose of 1.0 μM needed for a similar degree of inhibition (80%) in HepG2 cells. In contrast to the above report, simvastatin was found to decrease, rather than increase, apoB secretion (–31%), without affecting either apoB synthesis or apoB mRNA abundance. However, both cellular LDL receptor activity and mRNA abundance were increased by simvastatin treatment, at doses shown to inhibit cholesterol synthesis. These data suggest that competitive inhibition of HMG-CoA reductase by simvastatin triggered a coordinate regulation of genes coding for reductase and the LDL receptor, but not for apoB.

Using a rabbit hepatocyte culture system, Tanaka and colleagues treated cells with pravastatin to investigate the mechanisms that regulate apoB secretion in response to changes in intracellular CE content [33]. When cells were incubated with increasing concentrations of pravastatin (0.1–10 μg/mL), dose-dependent decreases in both *de novo* cholesterol synthesis and apoB secretion were observed, indicating that apoB secretion decreased in parallel with the decrease in cholesterolgenesis. Maximum inhibition of both apoB secretion and cholesterol synthesis was observed at a dose of 10 μg/mL, with values that were <40% and <5% of those for controls, respectively. Moreover, pravastatin, at a dose of 10 μg/mL, decreased the CE content of cells by 51%, without affecting cellular free cholesterol, phospholipid, or triglyceride concentrations.

Table 1. Selected *in vitro* studies performed during the past decade to examine the mechanisms by which statins reduce concentrations of apoB-containing lipoproteins

Reference	Statin	Cell Line(s)	Results	Conclusions
[31]	Simvastatin	Rat hepatocytes	Chol synthesis↓ ApoB synthesis & secretion↑ ApoB mRNA→	Simvastatin-induced ↑ in apoB synthesis occurred at the post-transcriptional level.
[32]	Simvastatin	HepG2 Human hepatocytes Rat hepatocytes	Chol synthesis↓ ApoB synthesis→ ApoB secretion↓ ApoB mRNA→	Simvastatin triggered a coordinate regulation of genes encoding for reductase and the LDL receptor but not for apoB.
[33]	Pravastatin	Rabbit hepatocytes	Chol synthesis↓ ApoB secretion↓ ApoB degradation↑ ApoB mRNA→	Pravastatin ↓ intracellular cholesteryl ester content which, in turn, leads to ↑ apoB degradation and, ultimately, ↓ apoB secretion.
[34]	Lovastatin	CaCo-2	Chol synthesis↓ ApoB secretion→	Despite inhibiting cholesterol synthesis, lovastatin did not alter apoB secretion.
[35]	Atorvastatin	HepG2	Chol synthesis↓ ApoB synthesis→ ApoB secretion↓ ApoB degradation↑ ApoB mRNA→	Atorvastatin alters apoB secretion and degradation primarily due to its inhibitory effect on cholesterol synthesis which, in turn, limits the availability of cholesterol for the normal assembly of lipoproteins.
[36]	Atorvastatin (A) Simvastatin (S)	HepG2	Chol synthesis (A↓, S↓) ApoB secretion (A↓, S↓)	Atorvastatin and simvastatin inhibited apoB secretion to a similar extent.
[37]	Atorvastatin Simvastatin	HepG2	Chol synthesis (A↓, S↓) ApoB synthesis (A→, S = ND) ApoB secretion (A↓, S→) ApoB degradation (A↑, S = ND) ApoB mRNA (A→, S→)	Atorvastatin, but not simvastatin, inhibits a pathway of apoB secretion that cannot be explained by differences in the extent of the inhibition of cholesterol synthesis.

The correlation between cellular CE content and apoB secretion was found to be 0.802, showing a positive, linear relationship between these two variables. Further analysis of the mechanisms responsible for the reduced apoB secretion revealed that this dose of pravastatin accelerated the intracellular degradation of apoB, without altering cellular apoB mRNA levels. These data suggest that intracellular CE content plays a critical role in apoB secretion, primarily by enhancing apoB degradation.

In 1995, Pau et al. reported the results of their study in which the possible role of cholesterol in regulating apoB secretion by the intestine was tested by suppression of cholesterol synthesis with lovastatin [34]. Differentiated post-confluent CaCo-2 cells were incubated for 24–72 h in the presence or absence of 5 μM lovastatin, and the secretion rates of lipids and apoproteins A-I and B were measured. At this dose, lovastatin markedly inhibited cholesterol synthesis in CaCo-2 cells for 48 h, with an increase in synthesis noted by the 72-h time point. Lovastatin also lowered intracellular CE content and reduced the rate of cholesterol secretion into the media. After stimulation of apoB secretion by the addition of 0.8 mM oleic acid to CaCo-2 cells, lovastatin was not found to inhibit apoB secretion during the first 48-h hour incubation period; however, by the 72-h time point, a 30% reduction in apoB secretion was observed. Their data further revealed that this reduction was not explained by an increase in the rate of LDL degradation. Based on these results, it can be concluded that the lovastatin-induced inhibition of cholesterol synthesis observed in this cell line did not significantly alter apoB secretion.

The effects of atorvastatin on the intracellular stability and secretion of apo B were investigated by Mohammadi and colleagues, using intact and permeabilized HepG2 cells [35]. Experiments were performed to examine the effects of atorvastatin on the: 1) rates of lipid synthesis and secretion, 2) synthesis and accumulation of apoB, 3) intracellular stability of apoB, 4) amount of apoB-containing lipoprotein particles assembled in HepG2 microsomes, and 5) secretion and accumulation of apoB into the culture medium. According to the authors' calculations, the doses of atorvastatin used in this study, 0.1 to 10 μmmol/L, closely related to plasma levels in patients treated with 10 to 80 mg of the drug. In a 70 kg man with a blood volume of 5 L, it was estimated that complete absorption of atorvastatin would result in a blood level of approximately 1.8 to 18 μmmol/L. Using pulse-labeling experiments with [^{3}H]acetate or [^{3}H]oleate, atorvastatin at this dose was found to inhibit the synthesis of cholesterol and CE but was not found to have a significant effect on either triglyceride or phospholipid synthesis. Atorvastatin was not determined to affect the synthesis of apoB; however, it significantly reduced apoB secretion (–28.5%) by enhancing apoB degradation and, furthermore, decreased the stability of apoB associated with lipoprotein particles. Based on these observations, it can be hypothesized that atorvastatin alters apoB secretion and degradation primarily as a result of its inhibitory effects on cholesterol synthesis which, in turn, limits the availability of cholesterol and/or CE for the normal assembly of apoB-containing lipoprotein particles.

In 1998, Bergstrom and colleagues reported the results of their studies in which the effects of atorvastatin and simvastatin on apoB secretion were compared [36]. In HepG2 cells treated with a broad range of either these statins (10 nM–10 μM), similar inductions of reductase activity, reductase protein, and reductase mRNA abundance were observed. When the ability of these statins to reduce apoB secretion was assessed, atorvastatin and simvastatin, each at a dose of 0.5 μM, inhibited apoB secretion to a similar extent (42% and 38%, respectively), leading these investigators to conclude that their data did not reveal any qualitative or mechanistic differences between these statins.

In contrast, Wilcox et al., who also compared the action of atorvastatin and simvastatin in the regulation of apoB secretion, reported that simvastatin had no effect on apoB secretion in the HepG2 cell system [37]. In these studies, atorvastatin at a dose of 10 μmmol/L significantly inhibited the synthesis of cholesterol by up to 96% and CE mass by 54%. Moreover, the accumulation of apoB in the media was reduced by 24% at a dose of 10 μmmol/L and by 36% at a dose of 20 μmmol/L. However, when compared with the same doses of atorvastatin, simvastatin was shown to have similar effects on cholesterol synthesis and CE mass but, conversely, was not found to have an effect on apoB secretion. Neither inhibitor affected apoB mRNA concentrations but both significantly increased LDL receptor and HMG-CoA reductase mRNA levels. To further characterize the reduction in apoB secretion observed with atorvastatin, pulse-chase experiments were performed and the resultant data were elaborately analyzed by multicompartmental modeling. These data revealed that atorvastatin did not affect the synthesis of apoB but, rather, decreased the secretion of apoB by 44% due to a proportionate increase in the intracellular degradation of apoB. The kinetics of apoB degradation were best described by including both rapid- and slow-turning over degradation compartments, with the effects of atorvastatin largely confined to the rapid compartment. These findings suggest that, in this cell system, atorvastatin, but not simvastatin, inhibits a pathway of apoB secretion via a mechanism that cannot be explained by differences in the extent of the inhibition of cholesterol synthesis.

In vivo *studies*

Early experiments designed to examine the effects of statin therapy on the metabolism of apoB-containing lipoproteins have yielded variable results. The metabolism of apoB-containing lipoproteins has been assessed in patients having a variety of primary hyperlipidemias, including heterozygous FH [11, 17], cholesteryl ester storage disease (CESD) [16], familial dysbetalipoproteinemia [10], and combined hyperlipidemia [8], as well as in those having a secondary hyperlipidemia such as that seen in nephrotic syndrome [18, 19]. Bilheimer and colleagues were the first to investigate the effects of a statin, mevinolin, on LDL kinetics [11]. In these studies, the statin-induced reductions in plasma cholesterol levels observed in six patients with heterozygous FH were attributed to increases in LDL receptor-mediated catabolism. Malmendier et al. similarly reported that treatment of seven normolipidemic subjects with simvastatin resulted in an increase in LDL receptor-mediated catabolism of apoB-containing lipoproteins [12]. Conversely, in twelve moderate hypercholesterolemic subjects treated with mevinolin, Grundy and colleagues observed that the reductions in LDL cholesterol were due to decreased production of LDL apoB, with no change noted in LDL fractional catabolic rate (FCR) [7]. Decreased production of LDL during statin therapy was also seen in one patient with CESD [16] and in three patients with nephrotic syndrome [18]. The reduced LDL apoB-100 production rates (PR) were the result of either increased uptake of very low density (VLDL) and/or intermediate density (IDL) lipoproteins or decreased secretion of apoB-containing lipoproteins by the liver. Finally, a study of lovastatin therapy in three subjects with familial dysbetalipoproteinemia demonstrated that both increased catabolism and decreased production of lipoproteins contributed to the observed reductions in LDL levels [10].

The results of *in vivo* kinetic studies performed during the past decade to examine the mechanisms by which statins reduce plasma concentrations of apoB-containing lipoproteins are summarized in Tables 2 and 3. Studies that employed radioactive tracers are presented in Table 2, whereas those that used stable isotope methodology are provided in Table 3. As can be seen in these tables, recent studies have also generated conflicting data, with respect to the kinetic mechanism(s) responsible for the LDL-lowering property of statins. Using ^{125}I-labeled VLDL and ^{131}I-labeled LDL, Arad et al. investigated the metabolism of VLDL, IDL, and LDL in seven patients with combined hyperlipidemia before and after lovastatin treatment (n = 2, 20 mg/qd; n = 5, 20 mg bid) [8]. Compared to baseline, treatment with lovastatin was associated with a significant reduction (–37%, $P < 0.003$) in the total rate of entry of apoB-containing lipoproteins into the plasma of all seven subjects. This reduction was attributed to decreases in VLDL and LDL apoB production rates, with no differences observed in either the percent conversion of VLDL to LDL or LDL apoB FCR. However, in three patients with FH, it was determined that lovastatin reduced LDL levels by increasing LDL apoB FCR.

In 1990, Vega, Krauss, and Grundy reported the results of their study that was designed to examine the effect of pravastatin on the metabolism of apoB in VLDL, IDL, and LDL in ten patients with primary moderate hypercholesterolemia [14]. After seven weeks, 20 mg bid of pravastatin reduced levels of cholesterol in VLDL, IDL, and LDL by 31%, 37%, and 29%, respectively, and decreased the apoB content of these particles as well. Using ^{131}I-VLDL as a tracer, it was revealed that these decreases were mainly due to a significant reduction in VLDL apoB PR (–40%), with a reduction in LDL apoB PR also noted in eight out of ten subjects. No changes were observed in VLDL, IDL, or LDL FCR. Analysis of LDL particle size, composition, and subclass pattern indicated that pravastatin did not produce consistent changes in these parameters. The findings indicate that, in these subjects, pravastatin acted by reducing

Table 2. *In vivo* kinetic studies performed during the past decade to examine the mechanisms by which statins reduce plasma concentrations of apoB-containing lipoproteins: radioisotope studies

Reference	Statin	Subjects	Method	Results	Conclusions
[8]	Lovastatin	Combined Hypercholesterolemia (n = 7);	^{125}I-VLDL ^{131}I-LDL	VLDL FCR → VLDL PR ↓ VLDL to LDL → LDL FCR → LDL PR ↓	
		FH (n = 3)		*LDL FCR* ↑ *LDL PR* →	↓LDL apoB due to reduced entry of apoB-containing lipoproteins into the plasma
[14]	Pravastatin	Moderate Hypercholesterolemia (n = 10)	^{131}I-$VLDL_1$	VLDL FCR → VLDL PR ↓ LDL FCR → LDL PR ↓	↓LDL-C due to ↓ input rate from VLDL and LDL via ↑ direct removal of nascent lipoproteins
[15]	Simvastatin	Moderate Hypercholesterolemia (n = 7)	^{131}I-$VLDL_1$ ^{125}I-$VLDL_2$	$VLDL_1$ direct uptake → $VLDL_2$ direct uptake ↑ $VLDL_{1+2}$ synthesis → $VLDL_1$ to $VLDL_2$ → $VLDL_2$ to IDL, LDL → IDL direct uptake ↑ IDL to LDL → LDL FCR →	↓LDL apoB PR due to ↑ direct catabolism of precursors
[38]	Lovastatin	Hyperlipidemia (n = 8)	^{131}I-C_1-LDL $^{125/131}$I-C_2-LDL $^{125/131}$I-Rx-LDL	LDL FCR ↑ LDL PR ↓	↓LDL-C due to ↑ LDL receptor activity, ↓ affinity of LDL for its receptor, and ↓ LDL apoB PR

C1 and C2, "control" LDL isolated during placebo phase; FCR, fractional catabolic rate; FH, familial hypercholesterolemia; PR, production rate; Rx, LDL isolated during statin phase.

Table 3. *In vivo* kinetic studies performed during the past decade to examine the mechanisms by which statins reduce plasma concentrations of apoB-containing lipoproteins: stable isotope studies

Reference	Statin	Subjects	Method	Results	Conclusions
[13]	Pravastatin	Mixed Hyperlipidemia (n = 5)	^{15}N-Glycine 1-^{13}C-Leucine	VLDL FCR ↑ LDL FCR ↑	↓ LDL levels due to ↑ FCR of apoB-containing lipoproteins
[17]	Simvastatin	Heterozygous FH (n = 6)	1-^{13}C-Leucine	VLDL SR ↓ LDL SR ↓ Mevalonic acid ↓	↓LDL-C associated with ↓ VLDL apoB secretion
[19]	Lovastatin	Nephrotic syndrome (n = 4)	1-^{13}C-Leucine	%VLDL to LDL ↓ LDL PR ↓	↓LDL PR due to ↓ conversion of VLDL to LDL via ↑ removal of VLDL from the plasma
[39]	Pravastatin	Familial combined hyperlipidemia (n = 5, from same kindred)	1-^{13}C-Leucine	VLDL FCR → VLDL PR → IDL FCR → IDL PR ↑ LDL FCR ↑ LDL PR → %VLDL to LDL →	↓ LDL levels due to ↑ FCR of both LDL-1 and LDL-2 subclasses
[40]	Lovastatin	Hyperlipidemia (n = 5)	$^{2}H_3$-Leucine	VLDL FCR → VLDL PR → or ↓ VLDL to IDL → IDL FCR → IDL PR ↓ IDL to LDL → LDL FCR → LDL PR ↓	
			$^{2}H_2O$	Chol FSR ↓ Chol PR ↓	↓IDL and LDL PR associated with ↓ *de novo* cholesterol synthesis

FCR, fractional catabolic rate; FH, familial hypercholesterolemia; PR, production rate; SR, synthesis rate

input rates of all apoB-containing lipoproteins, most likely due to enhanced removal of nascent lipoproteins and/or decreased synthesis of apoB by the liver.

Gaw and colleagues examined the effects of yet another statin, simvastatin, on the metabolism of apoB-containing lipoproteins in seven moderately hypercholesterolemic subjects [15]. Simvastatin therapy at a dose of 20 mg/day reduced LDL-C by 39% ($P < 0.001$), without altering either VLDL or HDL cholesterol concentrations. The effects of this statin on apoB metabolism were investigated using a dual tracer approach, in which $VLDL_1$ (Sf 60–400) and $VLDL_2$ (Sf 20–60) were radiolabeled with $I\text{-}^{131}$ and $I\text{-}^{125}$, respectively. $VLDL_1$ apoB pool size was unaltered by simvastatin therapy, as were its rates of synthesis, catabolism, and delipidation to $VLDL_2$. Although the pool size of $VLDL_2$ apoB was similarly unaltered, direct uptake of this particle was increased by simvastatin, as was the uptake of IDL. The 49% reduction ($P < 0.01$) in LDL apoB concentrations was primarily attributed to a decrease in synthesis. Thus, it appears that the reductions in LDL production rates reported in this study were a result of the increases observed in the direct uptake of $VLDL_2$ and IDL, with simvastatin having no effect on $VLDL_1$.

The most recent study to explore the role of statins in apoB metabolism using radiotracers is that of Berglund et al. [38]. In this study, the effects of lovastatin therapy, 40 mg/day, on LDL apoB metabolism were investigated in eight hyperlipidemic subjects (six males, two females), using a triple-tracer approach. LDL was isolated from subjects twice during the pretreatment phase, designated C_1-LDL and C_2-LDL, and once eight days after the initiation of lovastatin therapy, designated Rx-LDL. $^{131}I\text{-}C_1$-LDL was used for autologous LDL kinetic studies during the pretreatment phase, whereas C_2-LDL, isolated from plasma that had been stored at 4°C for eight days, and Rx-LDL were labeled with either I^{125} or I^{131} and injected into subjects. Using the latter tracers, it was observed that lovastatin caused a modest increase in LDL FCR (+21%, $P < 0.04$), with the increase in FCR being greater for the C_2-LDL tracer (+46%, $P < 0.02$). Additionally, LDL apoB PR decreased in seven of the eight subjects during lovastatin treatment, resulting in a mean reduction of 17% ($P < 0.03$). The relatively enhanced catabolism of LDL observed when pretreatment LDL, as opposed to on-treatment LDL, was used as a tracer was interpreted to indicate a decrease in the affinity of Rx-LDL for the LDL receptor. Thus, it can be concluded that lovastatin reduced plasma LDL levels in this study by increasing LDL receptor activity and decreasing LDL apoB PR, with a 15% decrease in affinity of LDL for its receptor partially negating the expected effect of increased LDL receptors on LDL clearance.

Table 3 summarizes the results of recent studies that have used stable isotope methodology to investigate the role of statins in apoB metabolism. In 1993, Parhofer et al. reported the results of their study that examined the effect of pravastatin on the metabolism of apoB in five men with mixed hyperlipoproteinemia [13]. Using a randomized, crossover design, kinetic parameters of apoB in subjects during placebo and pravastatin phases were determined by endogenous labeling with $1\text{-}^{13}C$-leucine and ^{15}N-glycine. Statin therapy reduced LDL cholesterol and LDL apoB levels by 20% and 29%, respectively. Multicompartmental modeling of the kinetic data revealed that these decreases were due to the combined effects of a 31% increase in VLDL apoB FCR ($P = 0.08$) and a 24% increase in LDL apoB FCR ($P < 0.01$), with apoB production rates remaining unchanged.

Using 1-^{13}C-leucine, Watts and colleagues studied the effects of eight weeks of simvastatin treatment (40 mg/day) on the metabolism of apoB-containing lipoproteins in six patients with heterozygous FH [17]. Simvastatin decreased plasma LDL cholesterol levels by 43% ($P = 0.002$) in these subjects, while increasing those of HDL cholesterol by 17% ($P = 0.02$). Moreover, a 20% reduction ($P = 0.002$) was seen in mevalonic acid levels, indicative of a decrease in cholesterol synthesis. Analysis of kinetic data showed that the absolute fractional secretion rate (ASR) of VLDL apoB was decreased by 83% and the fractional secretion rate (FSR) by 17% during simvastatin therapy. The change in the ASR of VLDL apoB was significantly correlated with the change in plasma LDL cholesterol concentration ($P < 0.04$), suggesting that the hepatic secretion of VLDL apoB was decreased by simvastatin in these FH patients.

Aguilar-Salinas et al. investigated the effects of lovastatin therapy on apoB metabolism in four men having a secondary hyperlipidemia due to nephrotic syndrome [19], in which there is both apoB over-production and accumulation of VLDL and LDL in the plasma. Endogenous labeling of apoB with 1-^{13}C-leucine and multicompartmental modeling were used to calculate the metabolic parameters of apoB-containing lipoproteins. After 6 weeks of treatment with lovastatin at 20 mg/day, significant reductions ($P < 0.01$) were noted in LDL cholesterol (–28%) and apoB (–18%) levels. Kinetic analysis revealed that lovastatin significantly decreased (–34%, $P = 0.03$) LDL apoB PR in all subjects. This was primarily due to the channeling of LDL precursors away from the LDL conversion pathway, as indicated by the 31% reduction ($P = 0.05$) seen in the percent of VLDL converted to LDL. Although the small number of subjects studied is a limitation of this work, these data are consistent with the concept that lovastatin decreases LDL levels in patients with nephrotic syndrome mainly by inhibiting the production of LDL from VLDL.

Aguilar-Salinas also examined the effects of pravastatin on apoB kinetics in five members of a kindred with familial combined hyperlipidemia (FCHL) [39]. This kindred differed somewhat from other FCHL kindreds in that decreased VLDL and LDL apoB clearance rates, rather than enhanced production rates, were the main kinetic abnormalities. ApoB metabolism was determined by endogenous labeling with 1-^{13}C-leucine, followed by multicompartmental modeling. After six weeks of treatment with 20 mg/day of pravastatin, no changes were seen in either VLDL apoB FCR or PR. Interestingly, IDL apoB PR was increased by 16% ($P < 0.03$), while IDL apoB FCR remained unchanged. The most dramatic difference noted between pre- and post-treatment values was the 79% increase ($P < 0.001$) in LDL apoB FCR. Analysis of LDL subfraction kinetics further revealed that this increase was due to enhanced catabolism of both LDL-1 (+61%) and LDL-2 (+68%), with LDL-1 cleared almost four times more rapidly than LDL-2. Thus, in this kindred, in whom catabolic defects caused FCHL, pravastatin reduced LDL cholesterol levels by increasing LDL apoB catabolism, rather than by decreasing LDL production.

In 1997, our laboratory reported the results of a study that examined the effects of lovastatin therapy on the metabolism of apoB-containing lipoproteins in the constantly fed state, as well as on the *de novo* synthesis of cholesterol, in five male subjects with combined hyperlipidemia [40]. Subjects were counseled to follow a Step 2 diet and were treated with placebo or lovastatin, 40 mg bid, in randomly assigned order for six-week periods. At the end of each experimental period, subjects were given deuterium oxide to assess *de novo* cholesterol synthesis and deuterated leucine to determine the kinetics of VLDL, IDL, and LDL apoB. Statin therapy resulted in significant reductions of LDL cholesterol (–27%) and LDL apoB (–16%) levels, while significant increases were noted in HDL cholesterol (+13%) and apoA-I (+11%) concentrations. Reductions were observed in both the FSR (–40%, $P = 0.04$) and PR (–42%, $P = 0.02$) of cholesterol. Lovastatin therapy did not affect VLDL, IDL, or LDL FCR, but it did decrease IDL apoB-100 PR by 31% ($P = 0.01$) and LDL apoB-100 PR by 35% ($P < 0.02$). From these data, we concluded that the decreased levels of LDL cholesterol observed after the treatment of combined hyperlipidemic subjects with lovastatin were due to decreases in *de novo* cholesterol synthesis and the PR of apoB-containing lipoproteins. The decline in *de novo* cholesterol synthesis, rather than an increase in the direct uptake of VLDL and IDL, may have contributed to the observed decline in production rates.

Effects on the metabolism of high density lipoproteins

Although the primary role of HMG-CoA reductase inhibitors is in the reduction of apoB-containing lipoprotein concentrations, several studies have shown that statins are also capable of increasing HDL cholesterol and apoA-I concentrations [40–45]. It has been demonstrated that these increases are due, in part, to statin-induced decreases in plasma CE transfer protein activity [46–48]. The most recent report on this subject is that of Guerin and colleagues [48]. These investigators observed that six weeks of treatment with atorvastatin at a dose of 10 mg/day significantly increased the relative proportion of HDL2a (+18%, $P < 0.004$), and decreased that of HDL3c (–10%, $P < 0.04$), in eighteen patients with combined hyperlipidemia, without altering total HDL mass. These changes were attributable to a decrease in CE transfer from HDL to the VLDL1 subfraction (–37%, $P = 0.006$), consequent to the reduction of VLDL1 concentrations caused by atorvastatin.

There is a paucity of data on the influence of statins on HDL metabolism. In fact, to our knowledge, the results of only two studies have been reported in the literature, one of which was in abstract form. In 1991, Ginsberg et al. presented the results of their study in which the effects of lovastatin on HDL kinetics were examined in seven subjects with isolated reductions of HDL cholesterol [49]. Lovastatin treatment increased plasma HDL cholesterol levels (mg/dL) by 5%, from a pre-treatment value of 31 ± 4 to a post-treatment value of 32 ± 5 ($P = 0.17$). A greater effect was observed on plasma apoA-I levels (mg/dL), with pre- and post-treatment values of 105 ± 28 and 124 ± 35 (+18%, $P < 0.05$), respectively. Kinetic studies, using ^{125}I-labeled HDL, revealed that apoA-I PR increased in four subjects, decreased in two subjects, and remained the same in one subject, resulting in a mean increase of 18% that was not statistically significant ($P = 0.24$) due to the variability observed between subjects. HDL apoA-I FCRs (pools/day) were unaffected by lovastatin, with a mean value of 0.28 ± 0.05 before lovastatin and of 0.28 ± 0.08 after. While these data suggest that lovastatin may increase HDL cholesterol levels by increasing apoA-I production and/or secretion, they are far from conclusive, especially in light of the fact that the increase in apoA-I PR seen in this study did not achieve statistical significance.

The most complete study described to date is that of Schaefer and colleagues [50]. This study was designed to examine the effects of pravastatin at a dose of 40 mg/day on the kinetics of HDL apoA-I in six normolipidemic males and one male CHD patient. HDL apoA-I kinetics were determined in all subjects both before and after treatment with pravastatin for a duration of 6 weeks. In the normolipidemic subjects, pravastatin increased plasma concentrations of HDL cholesterol by 13% and of apoA-I by 12%; however, these changes were not statistically significant due to the variable response of subjects. One subject experienced a 34% increase in HDL cholesterol, whereas another experienced a 2% reduction in HDL. The same was true of apoA-I, with one subject having a 30% increase in HDL cholesterol and another an 8% decrease.

In the one CHD patient studied, pravastatin reduced LDL and HDL cholesterol levels by 11% and 3%, respectively, and increased apoA-I by 2%. Using stable isotope methodology, it was determined that the mean FSR for apoA-I increased slightly (+5%) in normolipidemic subjects, indicative of enhanced catabolism of apoA-I, but increased to a greater extent in the CHD patient (+22%). In the former case, the elevated mean FSR value on pravastatin could be attributed solely to increases in three subjects, with this parameter remaining essentially unchanged in three others. Greater differences were observed in pre- and post-treatment values for apoA-I production rates. Four of the six normolipidemic subjects had an increase in apoA-I PR during treatment, resulting in a mean increase of 16% for this group. Similarly, the CHD patient also experienced an increase in apoA-I PR (mg/kg per day), with pre- and post-treatment values of 10.6 and 13.1 (+24%), respectively. From these data, the authors concluded that pravastatin mediates plasma HDL and apoA-I levels primarily by increasing apoA-I production rates. However, as was the case for the report by Ginsberg et al. [47], this conclusion is not entirely supported by their data, particularly in the CHD patient in whom apoA-I FSR and PR were affected to the same degree by pravastatin therapy, but in opposing directions. Due to the apparent heterogeneity in the HDL response of subjects to statin therapy, additional studies will be required before a more definitive statement on the role of this class of drugs in HDL metabolism can be made.

Conclusions

What is clear from the preceding studies is that statins significantly reduce concentrations of apoB-containing lipoproteins in the plasma. However, less clear is the mechanism(s) by which they do so. The majority of data from *in vitro* systems is consistent with the concept that statins reduce LDL apoB concentrations by decreasing intracellular cholesterol content which, in turn, increases apoB degradation and, ultimately, decreases apoB secretion. This translates into a reduction in the production of apoB-containing lipoproteins, as observed in a number of *in vivo* kinetic studies. To date, only two studies have carefully examined the role of statins in the regulation of HDL metabolism. Although they both suggest that statins increase HDL and apoA-I concentrations by increasing apoA-I production, the significant heterogeneity observed in the response of subjects in these studies makes it difficult to draw conclusions. Future experiments designed specifically to explore the role of various statins in HDL metabolism would be of great benefit.

References

1 The Expert Panel (1993) Summary of the report of the National Cholesterol Education Program Expert Panel on detection, evaluation, and treatment of high blood cholesterol in adults. *JAMA* 269: 3015–3023

2 American Heart Association (1998) 1998 heart and stroke statistical update. American Heart Association, Dallas, TX, B4

3 LaRosa JC, He J, Vupputuri S (1999) Effect of statins on risk of coronary heart disease: a meta-analysis of randomized controlled trials. *JAMA* 282: 2340–2346

4 Illingworth DR, Sexton GT (1984) Hypocholesterolemic effects of mevinolin in patients with heterozygous familial hypercholesterolemia. *J Clin Invest* 74: 1972–1978

5 Havel RJ, Hunninghake DB, Illingworth DR, Lees RS, Stein EA, Tobert JA, Bacon SR, Bolognese JA, Frost PH, Lamkin GE et al (1987) Lovastatin (mevinolin) in the treatment of heterozygous familial hypercholesterolemia: a multicenter study. *Ann Intern Med* 107: 609–615

6 The Lovastatin Group (1986) Therapeutic response to lovastatin (mevinolin) in nonfamilial hypercholesterolemia: a multicenter study. *JAMA* 256: 2829–2834

7 Grundy SM, Vega GL (1985) Influence of mevinolin on metabolism of low density lipoproteins in primary moderate hypercholesterolemia. *J Lipid Res* 26: 1464–1475

8 Arad Y, Ramakrishnan R, Ginsberg HN (1990) Lovastatin therapy reduces low density lipoprotein apoB levels in subjects with combined hyperlipidemia by reducing the production of apoB-containing lipoproteins: implications for the pathophysiology of apoB production. *J Lipid Res* 31: 567–582

9 Illingworth DR, O'Malley JP (1990) The hypolipidemic effects of lovastatin and clofibrate alone and in combination in patients with type III hyperlipidemia. *Metabolism* 39: 403–409

10 Vega GL, East C, Grundy SM (1988) Lovastatin therapy in familial dysbetalipo-proteinemia: effects on kinetics of apolipoprotein B. *Atherosclerosis* 70: 131–143

11 Bilheimer DW, Grundy SM, Brown MS, Goldstein JL (1983) Mevinolin and colestipol stimulate receptor-mediated clearance of low density lipoprotein from plasma in familial hypercholesterolemia heterozygotes. *Proc Natl Acad Sci USA* 80: 4124–4128
12 Malmendier CL, Lontie J-F, Delcroix C, Magot T (1989) Effect of simvastatin on receptor-dependent low density lipoprotein catabolism in normocholesterolemic human volunteers. *Atherosclerosis* 80: 101–109
13 Parhofer KG, Barrett PHR, Dunn J, Schonfeld G (1993) Effect of pravastatin on metabolic parameters of apolipoprotein B in patients with mixed hyperlipo-proteinemia. *Clin Invest* 71: 939–946
14 Vega GL, Krauss RM, Grundy SM (1990) Pravastatin therapy in primary moderate hypercholesterolemia: changes in metabolism of apolipoprotein B-containing lipoproteins. *J Intern Med* 227: 81–94
15 Gaw A, Packard CJ, Murray EF, Lindsay GM, Griffin BC, Caslake MJ, Vallance BD, Lorimer AR, Shepherd J (1993) Effects of simvastatin on apoB metabolism and LDL subfraction distribution. *Arterioscler Thromb* 13: 170–189
16 Ginsberg HN, Le N-A, Short MP, Ramakrishnan R, Desnick RJ (1987) Suppression of apolipoprotein B production during treatment of cholesteryl ester storage disease with lovastatin. *J Clin Invest* 80: 1692–1697
17 Watts GF, Cummings MH, Umpleby M, Quiney JR, Naoumova R, Thompson GR, Sonksen PH (1995) Simvastatin decreases the hepatic secretion of very-low-density lipoprotein apolipoprotein B-100 in heterozygous familial hypercholesterolaemia: pathophysiological and therapeutic implications. *Eur J Clin Invest* 25: 559–567
18 Vega GL, Grundy SM (1988) Lovastatin therapy in nephrotic hyperlipidemia: effects on lipoprotein metabolism. *Kidney Int* 33: 1160–1168
19 Aguilar-Salinas CA, Barrett PHR, Kelber J, Delmez J, Schonfeld G (1995) Physiologic mechanisms of action of lovastatin in nephrotic syndrome. *J Lipid Res* 36: 188–199
20 Marais AD, Naoumova RP, Firth JC, Penny C, Neuwirth CK, Thompson GR (1997) Decreased production of low density lipoprotein by atorvastatin after apheresis in homozygous familial hypercholesterolemia. *J Lipid Res* 38: 2071–2078
21 Raal FJ, Pilcher GJ, Illingworth DR, Pappu AS, Stein EA, Laskarzewski P, Mitchel YB, Melino MR (1997) Expanded dose simvastatin is effective in homozygous familial hypercholesterolemia. *Atherosclerosis* 135: 249–256
22 Endo A (2000) Discovery and development of the statins. *In*: A Gaw, CJ Packard, J Shepherd (eds): *Statins: the HMG CoA reductase inhibitors in perspective*. Martin Dunitz Ltd, London, 35–47
23 Endo A, Kuroda M, Tsujita Y (1976) ML-236A, ML-236B, and ML-236C: new inhibitors of cholesterolgenesis produced by *Penicillium citrinum*. *J Antibiot* (Japan) 29: 1346–1348
24 Endo A, Kuroda M, Tanzawa K (1976) Competitive inhibition of 3-hydroxy-3-methylglutaryl coenzyme A reductase by ML-236A and ML-236B, fungal metabolites having hypocholesterolemic activity. *FEBS Lett* 72: 323–326
25 Kaneko I, Hazama-Shimada Y, Endo A (1978) Inhibitory effects on lipid metabolism in cultured cells of ML-236B: a potent inhibitor of 3-methylglutaryl coenzyme A reductase. *Eur J Biochem* 87: 313–321
26 Gaw A, Packard CJ (2000) Comparative chemistry, pharmacology and mechanism of action of the statins. *In*: A Gaw, CJ Packard, J Shepherd (eds): *Statins: the HMG CoA reductase inhibitors in perspective*. Martin Dunitz Ltd, London, 49–61
27 Meadowcroft AM, Williamson KM, Patterson JH, Hinderliter AL, Pieper JA (1999) The effects of fluvastatin, a CYP2C9 inhibitor, on losartan pharmacokinetics in healthy volunteers. *J Clin Pharmacol* 39: 418–424
28 Anonymous (1994) Pravastatin (sodium). *In*: *Therapeutic Drug Supplements* 2. Churchill Livingstone, Edinburgh, 196–200
29 Muck W (1998) Rationale assessment of the interaction profile of cerivastatin supports its low propensity for drug interactions. *Drugs* 56 (suppl 1): 15–23
30 Azie NE, Brater DC, Becker PA, Jones DR, Hall SD (1998) The interaction of diltiazem with lovastatin and pravastatin. *Clin Pharmacol Ther* 64: 369–377
31 Ribeiro A, Mangeney M, Loriette C, Thomas G, Pepin D, Janvier B, Chambaz J, Bereziat G (1991) Effect of simvastatin on the synthesis and secretion of lipoproteins in relation to the metabolism of cholesterol in cultured hepatocytes. *Biochim Biophys Acta* 1086: 279–286
32 Qin W, Infante J, Wang S-R, Infante R (1992) Regulation of HMG-CoA reductase, apoprotein-B

and LDL receptor gene expression by the hypocholesterolemic drugs simvastatin and ciprofibrate in HepG2, human and rat hepatocytes. *Biochim Biophys Acta* 1127: 57–66

33 Tanaka M, Jingami H, Otani H, Cho M, Ueda Y, Arai H, Nagano Y, Doi T, Yokode M, Kita T (1993) Regulation of apolipoprotein B production and secretion in response to the change of intracellular cholesteryl ester contents in rabbit hepatocytes. *J Biol Chem* 268: 12,713–12,718

34 Pau E, He Y, Lougheed M, Steinbrecher UP (1995) Inhibition of hydroxymethylglutaryl coenzyme A reductase activity does not affect the secretion rate of apolipoproteins B and AI by CaCo-2 cells. *Biochem Cell Biol* 73: 81–90

35 Mohammadi A, Macri J, Newton R, Romain T, Dulay D, Adeli K (1998) Effects of atorvastatin on the intracellular stability and secretion of apolipoprotein B in HepG2 cells. *Arterioscler Thromb Vasc Biol* 18: 783–793

36 Bergstrom JD, Bostedor RG, Rew DJ, Geissler WM, Wright SD, Chao Y-S (1998) Hepatic responses to inhibition of 3-hydroxy-3-methylglutaryl-CoA reductase: a comparison of atorvastatin and simvastatin. *Biochim Biophys Acta* 1389: 213–221

37 Wilcox LJ, Barrett PHR, Huff MW (1999) Differential regulation of apolipoprotein B secretion from HepG2 cells by two HMG-CoA reductase inhibitors, atorvastatin and simvastatin. *J Lipid Res* 40: 1078–1089

38 Berglund L, Witzum JL, Galeano NF, Khouw AS, Ginsberg HN, Ramakrishnan R (1998) Threefold effect of lovastatin treatment on low density lipoprotein metabolism in subjects with hyperlipidemia: increase in receptor activity, decrease in apoB production, and decrease in particle affinity for the receptor. Results from a novel triple-tracer approach. *J Lipid Res* 39: 913–924

39 Aguilar-Salinas CA, Barrett PHR, Pulai J, Zhu XL, Schonfeld G (1997) A familial combined hyperlipidemic kindred with impaired apolipoprotein B catabolism: kinetics of apolipoprotein B during placebo and pravastatin therapy. *Arterioscler Thromb Vasc Biol* 17: 72–82

40 Cuchel M, Schaefer EJ, Millar JS, Jones PJH, Dolnikowski GG, Vergani C, Lichtenstein AH (1997) Lovastatin decreases *de novo* cholesterol synthesis and LDL apoB-100 production rates in combined-hyperlipidemic males. *Arterioscler Thromb Vasc Biol* 17: 1910–1917

41 Reihner E, Rudling M, Stahlberg D, Berglund L, Ewerth S, Bjorkhem I, Einarsson K, Angelin B (1990) Influence of pravastatin, a specific inhibitor of HMG-CoA reductase, on hepatic metabolism of cholesterol. *N Engl J Med* 323: 224–228

42 Jakob BG, Mohrle W, Richter WP, Schwandt P (1992) Short- and long-term effects of lovastatin and pravastatin alone and in combination with cholestyramine on serum lipids, lipoproteins and apolipoproteins in primary hypercholesterolemia. *Eur J Clin Pharmacol* 43: 353–358

43 The European Study Group (1992) Efficacy and tolerability of simvastatin and pravastatin in patients with primary hypercholesterolemia. *Am J Cardiol* 70: 1281–1286

44 The Simvastatin Pravastatin Study Group (1993) Comparison of the efficacy, safety, and tolerability of simvastatin and pravastatin for hypercholesterolemia. *Am J Cardiol* 71: 1408–1414

45 The Lovastatin Pravastatin Study Group (1993) A multicenter comparative trial of lovastatin and pravastatin in the treatment of hypercholesterolemia. *Am J Cardiol* 71: 810–815

46 Ahnadi CE, Berthezene F, Ponsin G (1993) Simvastatin-induced decrease in the transfer of cholesterol esters from high density lipoproteins to very low and low density lipoproteins in normolipidemic subjects. *Atherosclerosis* 99: 219–228

47 Guerin M, Dolphin PJ, Talussot C, Gardette J, Berthezene F, Chapman MJ (1995) Pravastatin modulates cholesteryl ester transfer from HDL to apoB-containing lipoproteins and lipoprotein subspecies profile in familial hypercholesterolemia. *Arterioscler Thromb Vasc Biol* 15: 1359–1368

48 Guerin M, Lassel TS, Le Goff W, Farnier M, Chapman MJ (2000) Action of atorvastatin in combined hyperlipidemia: preferential reduction of cholesteryl ester transfer from HDL to VLDL1 particles. *Arterioscler Thromb Vasc Biol* 20: 189–197

49 Ginsberg HN, Ngai C, Ramakrishnan R (1991) Lovastatin increases apoprotein A-I levels in subjects with isolated reductions in high density lipoproteins. *Circulation* 84: II-140 (abstract)

50 Schaefer JR, Schweer H, Ikewaki K, Stracke H, Seyberth HJ, Kaffarnik H, Maisch B, Steinmetz A (1999) Metabolic basis of high density lipoproteins and apolipoprotein A-I increase by HMG-CoA reductase inhibition in healthy subjects and a patient with coronary artery disease. *Atherosclerosis* 144: 177–184

Sterol-regulatory element binding proteins (SREBPs): gene-regulatory target of statin action

Jörg Kotzka[2], Wilhelm Krone[1] and Dirk Müller-Wieland[2]

[1] *Klinik II und Poliklinik für Innere Medizin der Universität zu Köln, D-50924 Köln, Germany*
[2] *Abteilung Klinische Biochemie und Pathobiochemie, Deutsches Diabetes-Forschungsinstitut an der Heinrich-Heine-Universität Düsseldorf, Auf'm Hennekamp 65, 40225 Düsseldorf, Germany*

Introduction: clinical perspectives of statin action

Several clinical studies have demonstrated over the last few years that efficient reduction of plasma cholesterol significantly reduces the incidence of clinical overt cardiovascular complications, like myocardial infarction or stroke, but has almost no effect on angiographically determined luminal diameter of coronary arteries. These, as well as many morphological and molecular studies, have led to a new paradigm of coronary heart disease, i.e., clinical prognosis is not mainly determined by the extent of a single stenosis, but by the number and biological nature of atherosclerotic plaques [1–7]. Considering biological and morphological features of atherosclerotic plaques, two types can be differentiated, stable and instable or vulnerable plaques. Vulnerable plaques are characterized by a large lipid-rich core with surrounding inflammation and a thin friable overlying fibrous cap susceptible to rupture or fissuring, thereby being a focus of high risk for thrombus formation. Rupture with consecutive thrombus formation can cause an acute coronary syndrome, such as unstable angina or myocardial infarction. So far reduction of plasma cholesterol by lipid-lowering therapy has been shown to reduce the lipid-rich core as well as inflammatory reactions, affect pro-coagulatory activity and increase extracellular matrix content and improve pardoxic vasocontriction by endothelial dysfunction. This might be due to efficient plasma cholesterol lowering and/or possible direct effects of statins on the vessel wall. Indeed, there is increasing evidence for the latter and therefore the concept that statins not only lower plasma cholesterol, but affect the biology of many cells, is carried even further. For example, besides cells within the vessel wall, statins appear to affect cells involved in inflammation, bone metabolism, lipid accumulation, and even insulin secretion like pancreatic β-cells [4, 6, 8]. This might lead to completely new research directions, for example, into the effect of statins on osteoporosis, obesity and possibly diabetes prevention. In this respect it is interesting to note that a recent *posthoc* analysis of the WOSCOP study indicates that, in the statin-treated group, incidence of overt type 2 diabetes was reduced by 30% [9]. This evidence implies that plasma cholesterol lowering by induction of the hepatic LDL receptor gene is only one effect of statin-mediated reduction of cholesterol synthesis in the liver. Besides induction of the LDL receptor gene, inhibition of HMG-CoA reductase by statins might affect the expression of many other genes and signaling pathways, e.g., those involved in reaction to stress and other extracellular stimuli, proliferation and apoptosis. As mentioned above, these so-called pleiotropic effects apparently have different implications for different cells and might lead to novel perspectives and clinical indications for statins in the near future.

Therefore, it is a current issue of research to understand the molecular mechanisms of how statins affect cell biology. There is no doubt that statins are competitive inhibitors of the key enzyme of cholesterol biosynthesis, i.e., the HMG-CoA reductase (see Fig. 1). The exact nature of statin binding to the enzyme has recently been shown by a crystallographic study [10]. If the activity of the key enzyme of cholesterol biosynthesis is reduced, one does not only reduce the endproduct of cholesterol synthesis, i.e., cholesterol, but also many intermediates, like farnesyl- and geranylgeranyl pyrophosphate, farnesyl and oxysterols. There is a growing body of evidence that cellular effects of statins are mediated by all of these molecular alterations related to inhibition of the cholesterol biosynthesis pathway. Lipid modifications like prenylation, i.e., post-translational modification of proteins by farnesyl pyrophosphate or geranylgeranyl pyrophosphate, regulate subcellular localizations of G-proteins, which affect many different signaling cascades within the cell. These mechanisms and their relation to statin action have been recently reviewed elsewhere [11, 12]. Another effect of inhibiting the cholesterol synthesis pathway is altering cellular gene expression by affecting the activity of nuclear orphan receptors, like FXR, OXR and LXR. Orphan receptors are transcription factors which are regulated by binding of metabolites, like farnesyl, oxysterols, and other lipids. In a recent review, these receptors were shown to play a pivotal role in the control of biliary cholesterol metabolism and cholesterol excretion, cholesterol uptake as well as foam cell formation [13, 14].

A different class of transcription factors which appear to be regulated by cholesterol has been identified by Brown and Goldstein [15]. Their group has asked the question: what is the cell biological signal within the cell linking intracellular cholesterol content to intranucleus events of inducing the LDL receptor gene? They have identified a cholesterol or sterol-sensitive sequence within the promoter region of the LDL receptor gene and isolated and characterized proteins interacting with this sequence, called sterol-regulatory element binding proteins (SREBPs). In the following we will review the structure and function of SREBPs and will provide a concept that they are targets of statins.

SREBPs: structure and function

There are three SREBP-isoforms, so-called SREBP-1a, SREBP-1c and SREBP-2, of which not only the human sequences but also the homologue

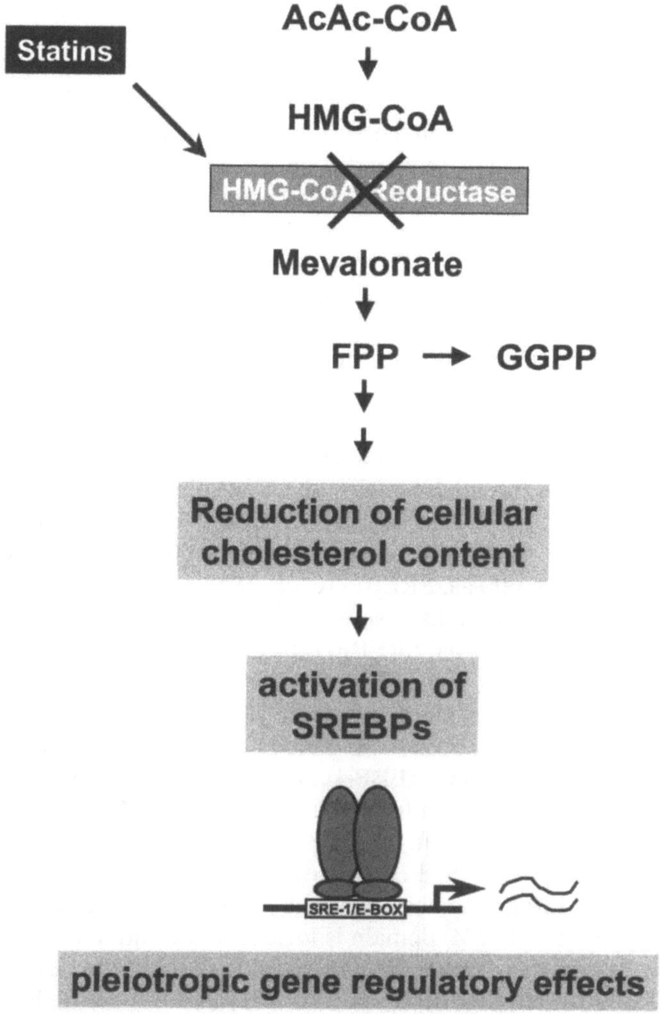

Figure 1. Molecular mechanisms for pleiotropic effects of statins. Inhibition of HMG-CoA reductase leads to a reduction of intermediates, like farnesyl pyrophosphate (FPP) and geranyl-geranylpyrophosphate (GGPP). These intermediates can regulate the activity of signalling cascades controlled by small G-proteins. Posttranslational lipid modification by these intermediates, also-called prenylation, control subcellular localization of some G-proteins, like Rho A. In addition, reduction of intracellular cholesterol content leads to an activation of cholesterol-regulated transcription factors, called sterol-regulatory element binding proteins (SREBPs). These transcription factors can regulate not only the expression of the LDL receptor gene, but also many others. Therefore, statin-mediated inhibition of cholesterol biosynthesis appears to affect a complex signalling and gene regulatory network which might be an explanation for the so-called "pleiotropic" statin effects. For further details, see text.

sequences of hamster and mice are known; SREBP-1 has also been sequenced from rat [16–21].

Gene and protein domain structure

Two of the three SREBP isoforms, SREBP-1a and SREBP-1c, are products of a single SREBP-1 gene [22–24]. They are generated by the recruitment of two distinct promotors and different first exons. Exon-1 of SREBP-1a codes for 29 amino acids, whereas SREBP-1c contains only 5 amino acids. These alternative exons are connected to a common second exon in the same reading frame by mRNA splicing. Although the chromosomal location of SREBPs (SREBP-1: 17p11.2, SREBP-2: 22q13) and gene sizes (SREBP-1: 26 kBp, SREBP-2: 72 kBp) are different, they apparently have a similar exon-intron structure, consisting of 19 exons [22, 23, 25]. Besides these mammalian proteins, helix loop helix (HLH) 106 has been isolated as a SREBP homologue in *Drosophila* [26, 27].

The SREBPs (SREBP-1a: 1147 aa, SREBP-1c: 1134 aa, SREBP-2: 1141 aa) have a sequence homology of 47% at the protein level [17]. The protein structure contains three essential domains, the N-terminal domain (SREBP-1a: ca. 460 aa, SREBP-1c: ca. 435 aa, SREBP-2: ca. 460 aa), two transmembrane domains containing a short loop of approximately 80 aa and a C-terminal domain (SREBP-1a: ca. 600 aa, SREBP-1c: ca. 585 aa, SREBP-2: ca. 600 aa). The N-terminal domain contains several regions beginning with a so-called acidic region (SREBP-1a: 51 aa, SREBP-1c: 27 aa, SREBP-2: 61 aa) exhibiting a sequence homology of 33%. This region is typical for transcription factors and appears to have a trans-activating role [28]. According to this hypothesis it has been shown that SREBP-1a, which contains a sequence 24 amino acids longer in this region than SREBP-1c, is a stronger activator of transcription [29]. This acid blob region is followed by a sequence which is rich in serine and proline residues, and in glycine in the case of SREBP-2. Then, SREBP-2, but not the two SREBP-1 isoforms, contains a glutamine-rich region; 27% of the 120 amino acid region are glutamine residues. The basic HLH leucin zipper (bHLH-LZ) domain is located at the end of the N-terminal domain. This region consists of 70 amino acids (SREBP-1a: aa 324–394, SREBP-1c: aa 300–370, SREBP-2: aa 331–401) and has the highest (71%) homology between the SREBPs. This domain contains three regions: the basic domain, the HLH domain and the leucin zipper domain. The basic domain appears to be a point of sequence-specific DNA protein interaction, whereas the HLH-LZ appears to be the region of dimerization mediating homo- or heterodimerization with other bHLH-proteins [30].

DNA binding motives and promoter studies

The family of bHLH-proteins consists of more than 400 different transcription factors which are important regulators in complex cellular networks, thereby playing a role in cell proliferation as well as cell differentiation, like neuro- and myogenesis [30–32]. All known bHLH-proteins bind to a palindromic

DNA sequence motive 5'-CANNTG-3', called E-box [33–35]. Further specifications lead to a classification of these transcription factors in four classes (A, B, C, and D) [31, 36–38]. Class A proteins bind to the recognition sequence 5'-CAGCTG-3' and proteins of class B recognize the sequence 5'-CACGTG-3'. Besides this hexanucleotide sequence, neighbouring nucleotides are also determining DNA binding of class C proteins. HLH transcription factors with a short basic domain, like ID, were classified separately (class D proteins), lacking transcriptional potency. Phylogenetic investigations provide evidence that class B proteins appear to be the oldest group [31, 38]. In accordance with that, transcription factors of this class have been found in all life-forms, whereas transcription factors of the other classes have been only identified in mammals.

The sterol-regulated element (sre)-1 in the promotor of LDL-receptor gene was identified as the original sterol-sensitive cis-element binding SREBPs. In contrast to the E-box motive, this element contains a direct base repeat (5'-ATCACCCCAC-3') [16, 39–42]. No other bHLH transcription factor binds to this motive. However, the group of Spiegelman has screened a rat adipocyte cDNA library using an oligonucleotide representing five repetitive E-box motives and found the rat homologue to SREBP-1c, called adipocyte determination- and differentiation factor (ADD)-1 [20]. They could show that ADD-1/SREBP-1c exhibits dual binding specificity, i.e., ADD-1/SREBP-1c cannot bind only to sre-1, but also to the E-box motive 5'-ATCACGTGA-3' [43]. In accordance with that, SREBPs can be classified as class B transcription factors. Additional studies show that a tyrosine residue in the basic domain of SREBPs appear to be responsible for the dual DNA binding specificity [43]. All other known bHLH transcription factors have an arginine residue in this position [30]. The exchange of tyrosine with arginine leads to a loss of SREBP-1 binding potency to sre-1 without affecting protein DNA interaction with the E-box sequence [43]. *Vice-versa*, substitution of the conserved arginine by a tyrosine in the bHLH-LZ transcription factor USF generated dual binding specificity [43]. Further evidence for dual binding specificity was derived from x-ray crystallographic investigations [44]. Co-crystallisation of SREBP-1a with sre-1 showed an almost symmetric homodimer with an asymmetric protein-DNA interaction. The monomer appears to bind to the half-site of E-box sequence (5'-ATCAC-3'), a protein-DNA interaction which has been also shown for the transcription factor Max [45]. Binding to the non E-box part within sre-1 (5'-GTGGG-3') is mediated via unknown contacts.

Previous studies have shown that promotors of many different genes contain a sre, with two direct repeats (5'-PyCAPy-3' [Py = pyrimidine]), separated by a nucleotide [46, 47]. However, there have been genes identified, which appear to contain a sre, which does not correspond to this consensus sequence [48–51]. The comparison of all known sres indicates that the nucleotide sequence to which SREBPs are binding exhibits no clear identifiable consensus sequence. This is in accordance with the hypothesis that the sre alone is not responsible for cholesterol-dependent transcriptional activation, but rather it depends on the interaction with other transcription factors, like NF-Y, SP1 or YY1 [48, 49, 52–73]. Furthermore, transcriptional activation appears to be dependent on the coactivator CREB-binding protein (CBP)/P300 or ARC [74–76].

Cholesterol-regulated control of intranuclear SREBP abundance

One essential difference of SREBP from known bHLH transcription factors is that SREBPs are embedded in the endoplasmatic reticulum, as well as in the nuclear envelope, as inactive precursors in a hairpin fashion [15, 77]. That means that the N-terminal and the C-terminal domains are interspaced by two membrane-spanning helices and one short loop localized in the lumen of the endoplasmatic reticulum or nuclear envelope.

Reduction of the intracellular sterol content leads to an enhanced release of the transcriptional active domain of the membrane-embedded SREBPs by activation of a proteolytic cascade [78]. This proteolytic cascade is initiated by a membrane-bound serine protease, called Site-1 protease (S1P), which cleaves SREBPs within the lumen of the endoplasmatic reticulum [79]. In SREBP-2 the enzyme cuts between leucine and serine within the amino acid sequence RSVLS [80]. For this S1P-mediated cleavage a basic amino acid in position 4, as well as leucine in position 1, is absolutely essential. All further positions do not contain a preference for any amino acid [80]. By this cleavage two peptide chains of the protein, which are inserted in the membrane, are generated [81]. After this initial cut the amino terminal domain is released by cleavage of a sterol-independent membrane-bound zinc metalloprotease, called site 2 protease (S2P) [82, 83]. In SREBP-2 this cleavage is between leucine and cysteine in the membrane-localized part of the sequence DRSRILLC, in which the second arginine appears to mark the border between the hydrophilic and hydrophobic sequence [83]. It has been shown that the tetra peptide DRSR is the recognition sequence for S2P; within the tetra peptide ILLC each amino acid can be changed to alanine without loss of function [83]. Meanwhile, this proteolytic mechanism of S2P, i.e., the capability to cut a protein within the membrane, has also been shown for other proteases. This has led to a proposal by Brown & Goldstein of the existence of a novel biological principle called regulated intramembrane proteolysis or Rip [84].

This proteolytical cascade is controlled by another protein, called SREBP cleavage-activating protein (SCAP) [85–87]. SCAP is an integral membrane protein (1276 aa) with eight membrane-spanning helices [88]. The N-terminal domain interacts with SREBPs and keeps the precursor proteins within the endoplasmatic reticulum. This association between SCAP and SREBPs is mediated by an interaction between the C-terminal regulatory domain of SREBPs with five WD-repeats within SCAP. Functional investigations showed that the formation of this complex is the precondition for S1P-mediated proteolysis; alterations of this complex generation by mutations in SREBP or SCAP prevents cleavage of membrane-embedded SREBPs [79, 89]. SCAP mediates the cleavage of SREBPs via a sterol-sensitive transmembrane domain and therefore appears to be a sensor of the intracellular cholesterol content [86]. Mutations of SCAP within this sterol-sensitive domain leads to a constitutively activated S1P-mediated release of SREBPs which is cholesterol-independent [86, 90, 91]. An analogous domain has been found in other cholesterol-regulated proteins [92–95]. Since the SCAP/SREBP complex is localized in the endoplasmatic reticulum and S1P is found in the post-endoplasmatic reticulum or Golgi apparatus, it is postulated that this subcellular separation is a key for the understanding of the cholesterol-dependent regulation of transcriptional active SREBPs [88, 91, 96–99]. Biochemical and genetic evidence has led to the model that SCAP actively transports SREBPs from the endoplasmatic reticulum to the post-endoplasmatic reticulum/Golgi apparatus and that this transport is reduced by cholesterol.

The SREBP precursor proteins are not only controlled by sterol-regulated proteolysis, but can also be a substrate of other proteases, e.g., SREBP cleavage activity (SCA-1) [100]. SCA-1 is the hamster homologue to the human protease CPP32, which again has a homology to the interleukin cleavage (converting) enzyme (ICE/CED-3) [101, 102]. SCA-1 releases the N-terminal domain of SREBP without the previous cholesterol-regulated luminal cut by a cleavage site which is close to but separate from the one belonging to S2P [100, 103]. Besides SCA-1, an additional protease has been identified (Mch3/SCA-2) which can release the N-terminal domain of SREBPs and which has a homology of 54% with CPP32/SCA-1 [104]. It is interesting to note that both proteins are cystein proteases, which have been related to apoptose cascades. Therefore it is a current issue of speculation whether SREBPs might play a role in apoptosis.

Gene targets of SREBPs

The released N-terminal domain of SREBPs containing the bHLH-LZ motive translocates via an interaction with importin-beta into the nucleus [105, 106], where the expression of target genes is regulated. A growing number of SREBP-regulated genes have been identified, which can be classified in five different groups: 1) Enzymes of cholesterol biosynthesis (HMG-CoA synthase, HMG-CoA reductase, farnesyldiphosphate synthase), 2) proteins involved in lipid catabolism (LDL receptor, lipoprotein lipase), 3) enzymes of fatty acid synthesis (acetyl-CoA carboxylase, fatty acid synthase, stearoyl-CoA desaturase 1, glycerol-3-phosphate acyltransferase), 4) regulators of intracellular transport (caveolin-1, caveolin-2) and 5) regulatory proteins (leptin) [46–49, 51–53, 56–59, 61, 62, 64, 65, 69, 72, 107–140].

Promoter studies show that cholesterol-regulated genes are activated via cis-elements of the sre-type and not via E-box sequences [141]. Therefore dual binding specifity of SREBPs appear to have a specific role [142]. In contrast to other bHLH transcription factors, SREBPs are mainly abundant as transcription factors within the nucleus after release from precursor proteins by reduction of intracellular cholesterol content. If cholesterol-regulated genes would also be regulated by cis-elements of the E-box type, other transcription factors of the bHLH family could activate them. This would lead to a rather independent regulation of these target genes. Therefore the sterol-regulated cis-element of the sre-type appears to make sure that target genes are only activated to be adaptive to the modulation of the intracellular cholesterol content. However, since SREBPs are also capable of binding to cis-elements of the E-box type, lipid-controlled gene regulatory signaling is spread and converges with other cellular signaling pathways at these elements. Thereby, for example, the dual specificity of SREBPs leads not only to regulation of cholesterol, but also lipid, synthesis.

Pathophysiological phenomena in mice with altered SREBP abundance

Many investigations, mainly in transgenic mice, indicate that SREBP-1a and SREBP-1c regulate predominantly fatty acid metabolism and *de novo* synthesis, whereas SREBP-2 appears to be the master regulator of cholesterol homeostasis [24, 29, 143–147]. Transgenic mice overexpressing the N-terminal domain of SREBP-1a under the control of the phosphoenolpyruvate-carboxykinase (PEPCK) promoter exhibit a 4-fold increase of the liver size after a protein-rich diet. This is the consequence of an increased accumulation of cholesterol and triglycerides [144]. Cholesterol synthesis increased 5-fold and fatty acid synthesis by 25-fold in the liver of these animals, whereas the concentration of plasma lipids was unaltered. Only crossing of these mice with LDL receptor knock-out mice led to a dramatic increase of plasma lipids [148]. From these observations it was concluded, that the lack of increase in plasma lipids in SREBP-1a-overexpressing animals was due to a dramatic upregulation of the hepatic LDL receptor. Overexpression of SREBP-1c led only to an increase of liver size of 33% [29]. The triglyceride content was slightly increased but the cholesterol content was unaltered. Transgenic mice overexpressing the transactive domain of SREBP-2 under the PEPCK promoter showed a 28-fold increase of cholesterol synthesis, but only a 4-fold stimulation of fatty acid synthesis [146]. Further experiments with these three transgenic mice models indicate a dominant role of SREBP-1 in the regulation of enzymes involved in lipid metabolism, whereas SREBP-2 appears to play a dominant role in the regulation of cholesterol metabolism [149]. Feeding experiments showed that there appears to be a relation between the nutrition, SREBP-regulation and fatty acid and cholesterol metabolism [145]. Further insights into the differential function of SREBP isoforms were obtained by knock-out mice [150]. 50–85% of SREBP-$1^{-/-}$ knock-out mice died within in the uterus at the 11th day of gestation. However, survivors had a normal phenotype. In these animals SREBP-2 was increased 1.5-fold at the mRNA level and at the protein level there was a 2–3-fold upregulated content in the nuclei of liver. Cholesterol biosynthesis was increased 3-fold and the cholesterol content of liver was elevated by 50%. Fatty acid synthesis, however, was only decreased by 40%. This might be due to a potential compensatory role of SREBP-2 or a yet unknown factor might exist which can compensate for the loss of SREBP-1. In contrast to that, SREBP-2 knock-out mice are completely lethal in a very early developmental stage.

Spiegelman's group could show that ADD-1/SREBP-1c plays an essential role in adipocyte differentiation [20, 151]. Ectopic expression of ADD-1/SREBP-1c in 3 T3-L1 pre-adipocytes led to a dramatic increase in differentiation markers, like expression of adipocyte protein (aP)2, lipoprotein lipase (LPL), peroxisome proliferator activator receptor (PPAR)γ2 and CAAT/enhancer binding protein (C/EBP) [151–153]. Although SREBP-1a appears to be the predominant isoform in different cell culture experiments [24], SREBP-1c appears to be the predominant isoform in white adipose tissue of mice and men [24, 152]. Ectopic expression of a negative form of ADD-1/SREBP-1c prevents the differentiation of 3 T3-L1 pre-adipocytess into adipocytes [151]. In contrast to that, the expression of the wild type activates genes which are involved in fat cell differentiation and lipid accumulation. In this process, ADD-1/SREBP-1c appears to cooperate with the nuclear receptor PPARγ2, which is the essential transcription factor of adipocyte differentiation [151, 154–158]. Under addition of a PPARγ2 activator to pre-adipocytes, about 2–3% of the cells differentiate into adipocytes. Transfection of the cells with ADD-1/SREBP-1c enhances the effect of PPARγ2 activators dramatically, i.e., 15–20% of pre-adipocytes differentiate into adipocytes. This cooperative act appears to be related to ADD-1/SREBP-1c-dependent generation of endogenous PPARγ2 ligands [159]. Additional experiments have led to the hypothesis that ADD-1/SREBP-1c not only plays a role in adipocyte differentiation, but also in the nutritional and hormonal control of genes involved in lipid metabolism and leptin signaling [152]. Transgenic mice overexpressing SREBP-1a in the liver not only have massive lipid accumulation in this organ, but also a dramatic reduction of white adipose tissue [144]. In transgenic mice overexpressing ADD-1/SREBP-1c in the liver, this reduction in white adipose tissue was not observed [29]. However, animals overexpressing ADD-1/SREBP-1c in adipocytes by using the aP2 promoter, lack fat tissue [149, 160]. Interestingly, these animals develop severe insulin resistance with hyperglycaemia and hypertriglyceridaemia, resembling the clinical picture of generalized lipodystrophy [161, 162]. Further evidence that SREBPs are required for cellular lipid synthesis and are targets of insulin action has been obtained by a mice model, in which the SREBP cleavage-activating protein (SCAP) has been conditionally deleted in the liver [163]. These liver-specific SCAP-deficient mice exhibit an 80% reduction in the basal synthesis rates of cholesterol as well as fatty acids and blunted gene regulatory responses to cholesterol deprivation, fasting and refeeding.

SREBPs: mediators of statin action?

There are increasing data that SREBPs modulate and mediate effects of statins and *vice-versa*, that statins affect the abundance of SREBPs. In case intracellullar cholesterol-lowering with consecutive induction of the LDL receptor gene by competitive inhibition of the key regulatory enzyme in cholesterol synthesis, HMG-CoA reductase, is the sole mechanism of statins, one would expect that this gene-regulatory event is mediated by SREBPs (see Fig. 1). In contrast to that, in our SREBP-1-deficient hepatoma cell lines the effect of statins on the LDL receptor promotor was not affected [164], but even increased several-fold in SREBP-2-deficient cells (Kotzka J et al., unpublished data). In accordance with that, overexpressing the corresponding SREBPs decreased the effects of statins on the LDL receptor gene. These data show that the intracellular abundance of SREBPs modulates the effectivity of statins. This might be a molecular mechanism explaining why there are different responses of statin-induced LDL cholesterol-lowering in plasma between individuals. However, proof of principle that SREBPs mediate statin action was obtained in cells that were deficient in both SREBP-1 and SREBP-2. In these cell lines, the effect of statins on LDL receptor promotor activity was completely abolished (Kotzka J et al., unpublished data). Accordingly, in liver-specific SCAP-deficient mice exhibiting reduced SREBP-cleavage capacity, the gene-regulatory response to statins was blunted [163].

On the other hand, statins appear to affect the expression levels of SREBPs. Animals treated with a combination of a bile acid-binding resin and the statin mevinolin indicate that SREBPs are differentially regulated by statins. In hamsters it has been shown that statin treatment increased the amount of SREBP-2 in the liver and decreased the mRNA and protein levels of SREBP-1c [165].

Interestingly, using a cultured rat hepatoma cell line mimicking the behavior of SREBP expression of rat liver, it has been shown that the high level of SREBP-1c mRNA is abolished when cholesterol synthesis is blocked by a statin [166]. This effect is reversible by mevalonate and by liver X receptor (LXR) ligands. In accordance with that, it has been shown recently that the mouse SREBP-1c gene is regulated by the LXRs which belong to the nuclear hormone receptor superfamily and are activated by oxysterols [167, 168]. SREBP-1c expression is increased by dietary cholesterol in a LXR-dependent manner; an effect which is antagonized by unsaturated fatty acids [169]. Since SREBP-1c plays a predominant role compared to SREBP-2 in the induction of fatty acid synthesis, this mechanism seems to be a gene-regulatory link between dietary cholesterol and fatty acid synthesis.

SREBPs: a gene-regulatory link for different cardiovascular risk factors

Gene regulation determines the abundance of proteins which are central players in the metabolism, differentiation and growth of cells. Therefore, alterations in gene regulation can have pleiotropic effects in the pathophysiology of multifactorial diseases, like atherosclerosis and cardivascular risk factors. Cardiovascular risk factors, like arterial hypertension, obesity, diabetes mellitus type 2 or glucose intolerance, and disorders of lipid metabolism, are multifactorial polygenic diseases, which are frequently found in a single individual. This clinical clustering of cardiovascular risk factors appears to be associated with decreased insulin sensitivity or insulin resistance. Therefore one current hypothesis is that mechanisms might exist at the molecular level linking decreased insulin sensitivity with the development of these coronary risk factors. Transcription factors are such candidates, because they regulate the expression of many genes and are targets of different intracellular signaling cascades, coupling stimuli from the cell surface to gene-regulatory events. Well-known examples are PPARs and SREBPs, integrating signals from metabolites and hormones at a gene-regulatory level. PPARs, for example, play an essential role in the control of lipid metabolism, insulin sensitivity and adipocyte differentiation and are targets of drugs used in the treatment of lipid disorders, i.e., fibrates (PPARα), and in the control of blood glucose levels, i.e., glitazones (PPARγ) [13, 170, 171]. Just recently, first evidence has been provided that there might be a cross-talk between statins and fibrates, because statins can induce the apolipoprotein A1 gene promoter via PPARα [172].

One interesting aspect arising at the pathophysiological level is that increased intracellular lipid accumulation might impair the function of the corresponding cell, e.g., insulin sensitivity in the case of adipose tissue, skeletal muscle and liver. In this respect, intracellular lipid accumulation, called lipid toxicity, might be a link between insulin resistance, obesity and increased lipid deposition in non-adipose tissue, possibly including cells of the arterial vessel wall [173–177]. Apparently SREBPs are key players in the control of intracellular lipid accumulation. Therefore, also in this regard it is interesting to note that SREBPs might not only be targets of statins, but also appear to be a gene-regulatory point of convergence between intracellular cholesterol as well as fatty acid homeostasis and other features linking insulin resistance, obesity, and possible atherosclerosis.

Conclusion

SREBPs are a novel protein family which appear to play an essential role in molecular signaling mechanisms of cholesterol lowering. They are new intracellular mediators linking metabolic alterations to gene regulatory events, some of which might play an important part in the concert of plaque biology. Who knows, perhaps SREBPs built the bridge between dyslipidemia and other cardiovascular risk factors like obesity and the syndrome of insulin resistance.

References

1 Müller-Wieland D, Kotzka J, Krone W (1997) Stabilization of atherosclerotic plaque during lipid lowering. *Curr Opin Lipidol* 8: 348–353

2 Rosenson RS, Tangney CC (1998) Antiatherothrombotic properties of statins: implications for cardiovascular event reduction. *JAMA* 279: 1643–1650

3 Ravn HB, Falk E (1999) Histopathology of plaque rupture. *Cardiol Clin* 17: 263–170

4 Rosenson RS (1999) Non-lipid-lowering effects of statins on atherosclerosis. *Curr Cardiol Rep* 1: 225–232

5 Adams MR, Kinlay S, Blasé GJ, Orford JL, Ganz P, Selwyn AP (2000) Pathophysiology of atherosclerosis: development, regression, restenosis. *Curr Atheroscler Rep* 2: 251–258

6 Farmer JA (2000) Pleiotropic effects of statins. *Curr Atheroscler Rep* 2: 208–217

7 Libby P (2000) Coronary artery injury and the biology of atherosclerosis: inflammation, thrombosis, and stabilization. *Am J Cardiol* 86 (8 Suppl 2): 3–8

8 Laudes M, Kotzka J, Avci H, Rastalsky N, Krone W, Müller-Wieland D (2001) Effect of glucose on sterol regulatory element binding protein (SREBP)-1 in pancreatic beta cells. *Diabetes* 50 (Suppl. 2): A354

9 Freeman DJ, Norrie J, Sattar N, Neely RD, Cobbe SM, Ford I, Isles C, Lorimer AR, Macfarlane PW, McKillop JH et al (2001) Pravastatin and the development of diabetes mellitus: evidence for a protective treatment effect in the West of Scotland Coronary Prevention Study. *Circulation* 103: 357–462

10 Istvan ES, Planitkar M, Buchanan SK, Deisenhofer J (2000) Crystal structure of the catalytic portion of human HMG-CoA reductase: insights into regulation of activity and catalysis. *EMBO J* 19: 819–830

11 Hughes AD (1996) The role of isoprenoids in vascular smooth muscle: potential benefits of statins unrelated to cholesterol lowering. *J Hum Hypertens* 10: 387–390

12 Edwards PA, Ericsson J (1999) Sterols and isoprenoids: Signaling molecules derived from the cholesterol biosynthetic pathway. *Annu Rev Biochem* 68: 157–185

13 Auwerx J, Mangelsdorf D (2000) X-ceptors, nuclear receptors for metabolism. *In*: S Stemme, AG Olsson (eds): *Atherosclerosis XII*. Elsevier Science B. V., Amsterdam, 21–39

14 Fayard E, Schoonjans K, Auwerx J (2001) Xol INXS: role of the liver X and the farnesol X receptors. *Curr Opin Lipidol* 12: 113–120

15 Brown MS, Goldstein JL (1997) The SREBP pathway: regulation of cholesterol metabolism by proteolysis of a membrane-bound transcription factor. *Cell* 89: 331–340

16 Briggs MR, Yokoyama C, Wang X, Brown MS, Goldstein JL (1993) Nuclear protein that binds sterol regulatory element of low density lipoprotein receptor promoter. I. Identification of the protein and delineation of its target nucleotide sequence. *J Biol Chem* 268: 14490–14496

17 Wang X, Briggs MR, Hua X, Yokoyama C, Goldstein JL, Brown MS (1993) Nuclear protein that binds sterol regulatory element of low density lipoprotein receptor promoter. II. Purification and characterization. *J Biol Chem* 268: 14497–14504

18 Wang X, Sato R, Brown MS, Hua X, Goldstein JL (1994) SREBP-1 a membrane-bound transcription factor released by sterol-regulated proteolysis. *Cell* 77: 53–62

19 Hua X, Yokoyama C, Wu J, Briggs MR, Brown MS, Goldstein JL, Wang X (1993) SREBP-2, a second basic-helix-loop-helix-leucine zipper protein that stimulates transcription by binding to a sterol regulatory element. *Proc Natl Acad Sci USA* 90: 11603–11607

20 Tontonoz P, Kim JB, Graves RA, Spiegelman BM (1993) ADD1: a novel helix-loop-helix transcription factor associated with adipocyte determination and differentiation. *Mol Cell Biol* 13: 4753–4759

21 Sato R, Yang J, Wang X, Evans MJ, Ho YK, Goldstein JL, Brown MS (1994) Assignment of the membrane attachment, DNA binding, and transcriptional activation domains of sterol regulatory element-binding protein-1 (SREBP-1). *J Biol Chem* 269: 17267–17273

22 Yokoyama C, Wang X, Briggs MR, Admon A, Wu J, Hua X, Goldstein JL, Brown MS (1993) SREBP-1, a basic-helix-loop-helix-leucine zipper protein that controls transcription of the low density lipoprotein receptor gene. *Cell* 75: 187–197

23 Hua X, Wu J, Goldstein JL, Brown MS, Hobbs HH (1995) Structure of the human gene encoding sterol regulatory element binding protein-1 (SREBP1) and localization of SREBP1 and SREBP2 to chromosomes 7p11.2 and 22q13. *Genomics* 25: 667–673

24 Shimomura I, Shimano H, Horton JD, Goldstein JL, Brown MS (1997) Differential expression of exons 1a and 1c in mRNAs for sterol regulatory element binding protein-1 in human and mouse organs and cultured cells. *J Clin Invest* 99: 838–845
25 Miserez AR, Cao G, Probst LC, Hobbs HH (1997) Structure of the human gene encoding sterol regulatory element binding protein 2 (SREBP2). *Genomics* 40: 31–40
26 Theopold U, Ekengren S, Hultmark D (1996) HLH106, a *Drosophila* transcription factor with similarity to the vertebrate sterol responsive element binding protein. *Proc Natl Acad Sci USA* 93: 1195–1199
27 Rosenfeld JM, Osborne TF (1998) HLH106, a *Drosophila* sterol regulatory element-binding protein in a natural cholesterol auxotroph. *J Biol Chem* 273: 16112–16121
28 Ma J, Ptashne M (1987) A new class of yeast transcriptional activators. *Cell* 51: 113–119
29 Shimano H, Horton JD, Shimomura I, Hammer RE, Brown MS, Goldstein JL (1997) Isoform 1c of sterol regulatory element binding protein is less active than isoform 1a in livers of transgenic mice and in cultured cells. *J Clin Invest* 99: 846–854
30 Littlewood TD, Evan GI (1995) Transcription factors 2: helix-loop-helix. *Protein Profile* 2: 621–702
31 Morgenstern B, Atchley WR (1999) Evolution of bHLH transcription factors: modular evolution by domain shuffling? *Mol Biol Evol* 16: 1654–1663
32 Massari ME and Murre C (2000) Helix-loop-helix proteins: regulators of transcription in eucaryotic organisms. *Mol Cell Biol* 20: 429–440
33 Murre C, McCaw PS, Baltimore D (1989) A new DNA binding and dimerization motif in immunoglobulin enhancer binding, daughterless, Myo D, and myc proteins. *Cell* 56: 777–783
34 Voronova A, Baltimore D (1990) Mutations that disrupt DNA binding and dimer formation in the E47 helix-loop-helix protein map to distinct domains. *Proc Natl Acad Sci USA* 87: 4722–4726
35 Murre C, Baltimore D (1992) *In*: SL McKnight and Yamamoto (eds): *Transcriptional Regulaton.* K.R. Cold Spring Harbor Laboratory Press, Plainview, New York, 861–879
36 Deng CV, Dolde C, Gillison ML, Kato GJ (1992) Discrimination between related DNA sites by a single amino acid residue of Myc-related basic-helix-loop-helix proteins. *Proc Natl Acad Sci USA* 89: 599–602
37 Swanson HI, Chan WK, Bradfield CA (1995) DNA binding specificities and pairing rules of the Ah receptor, ARNT, and SIM proteins. *J Biol Chem* 270: 26292–26302
38 Atchley WR, Fitch WM (1997) A natural classification of the basic helix-loop-helix class of transcription factors. *Proc Natl Acad Sci USA* 94: 5172–5176
39 Südhof TC, Russell DW, Goldstein JL, Brown MS, Sanchez-Pescador R, Bell GI (1985) Cassette of eight exons shared by genes for LDL receptor and EGF precursor. *Science* 228: 893–895
40 Südhof TC, Goldstein JL, Brown MS, Russell DW (1985) The LDL receptor gene: a mosaic of exons shared with different proteins. *Science* 228: 815–822
41 Südhof TC, Russell DW, Brown MS, Goldstein JL (1987) 42 bp element from LDL receptor gene confers end-product repression by sterols when inserted into viral TK promoter. *Cell* 48: 1061–1069
42 Südhof TC, van der Westhuyzen DR, Goldstein JL, Brown MS, Russell DW (1987) Three direct repeats and a TATA-like sequence are required for regulated expression of the human low density lipoprotein receptor gene. *J Biol Chem* 262: 10773–10779
43 Kim JB, Spotts GD, Halvorsen YD, Shih HM, Ellenberger T, Towle HC, Spiegelman BM (1995) Dual DNA binding specificity of ADD1/SREBP1 controlled by a single amino acid in the basic helix-loop-helix domain. *Mol Cell Biol* 15: 2582–2588
44 Parraga A, Bellsolell L, Ferré-D'Amaré AR, Burley SK (1998) Co-crystal structure of sterol regulatory element binding protein 1a at 2.3 Å resolution. *Structure* 6: 661–672
45 Ferré-D'Amaré AR, Prendergast GC, Ziff EB, Burley SK (1993) Recognition by Max of its cognate DNA trough a dimeric b/HLH/Z domain. *Nature* 363: 38–45
46 Magana MM, Osborne TF (1996) Two tandem binding sites for sterol regulatory element binding proteins are required for sterol regulation of fatty-acid synthase promoter. *J Biol Chem* 271: 32689–32694
47 Magana MM, Lin SS, Dooley KA, Osborne TF (1997) Sterol regulation of acetyl coenzyme A carboxylase promoter requires two interdependent binding sites for sterol regulatory element binding proteins. *J Lipid Res* 38: 1630–1638
48 Ericsson J, Jackson SM, Lee BC, Edwards PA (1996) Sterol regulatory element binding protein binds to a cis element in the promoter of the farnesyl diphosphate synthase gene. *Proc Natl Acad*

Sci USA 93: 945–950
49 Ericsson J, Jackson SM, Kim JB, Spiegelman BM, Edwards PA (1997) Identification of glycerol-3-phosphate acyltransferase as an adipocyte determination and differentiation factor 1- and sterol regulatory element-binding protein-responsive gene. *J Biol Chem* 272: 7298–7305
50 Guan G, Dai P, Shechter I (1998) Differential transcriptional regulation of the human squalene synthase gene by sterol regulatory element-binding proteins (SREBP) 1a and 2 and involvement of 5' DNA sequence elements in the regulation. *J Biol Chem* 273: 12526–12535
51 Tabor DE, Kim JB, Spiegelman BM, Edwards PA (1998) Transcriptional activation of the stearoyl-CoA desaturase 2 gene by sterol regulatory element-binding protein/adipocyte determination and differentiation factor 1. *J Biol Chem* 273: 22052–22058
52 Bennett MK, Lopez JM, Sanchez HB, Osborne TF (1995) Sterol regulation of fatty acid synthase promoter. Coordinate feedback regulation of two major lipid pathways. *J Biol Chem* 270: 25578–25583
53 Guan G, Jiang G, Koch RL, Shechter I (1995) Molecular cloning and functional analysis of the promoter of the human squalene synthase gene. *J Biol Chem* 270: 21958–21965
54 Sanchez HB, Yieh L, Osborne TF (1995) Cooperation by sterol regulatory element-binding protein and Sp1 in sterol regulation of low density lipoprotein receptor gene. *J Biol Chem* 270: 1161–1169
55 Yieh L, Sanchez HB, Osborne TF (1995) Domains of transcription factor Sp1 required for synergistic activation with sterol regulatory element binding protein 1 of low density lipoprotein receptor promoter. *Proc Natl Acad Sci USA* 92: 6102–6106
56 Ericsson J, Jackson SM, Edwards PA (1996) Synergistic binding of sterol regulatory element-binding protein and NF-Y to the farnesyl diphosphate synthase promoter is critical for sterol-regulated expression of the gene. *J Biol Chem* 271: 24359–24364
57 Jackson SM, Ericsson J, Metherall JE, Edwards PA (1996) Role for sterol regulatory element binding protein in the regulation of farnesyl diphosphate synthase and in the control of cellular levels of cholesterol and triglyceride: evidence from sterol regulation-defective cells. *J Lipid Res* 37: 1712–1721
58 Lopez JM, Bennett MK, Sanchez HB, Rosenfeld JM, Osborne TE (1996) Sterol regulation of acetyl coenzyme A carboxylase: a mechanism for coordinate control of cellular lipid. *Proc Natl Acad Sci USA* 93: 1049–1053
59 Sato R, Inoue J, Kawabe Y, Kodama T, Takano T, Maeda M (1996) Sterol-dependent transcriptional regulation of sterol regulatory element-binding protein-2. *J Biol Chem* 271: 26461–26464
60 Athanikar JN, Sanchez HB, Osborne TF (1997) Promoter selective transcriptional synergy mediated by sterol regulatory element binding protein and Sp1: a critical role for the Btd domain of Sp1. *Mol Cell Biol* 17: 5193–5200
61 Dooley KA, Millinder S, Osborne TF (1998) Sterol regulation of 3-hydroxy-3-methylglutaryl-coenzyme A synthase gene through a direct interaction between sterol regulatory element binding protein and the trimeric CCAAT-binding factor/nuclear factor Y. *J Biol Chem* 273: 1349–1356
62 Inoue J, Sato R, Maeda M (1998) Multiple DNA elements for sterol regulatory element-binding protein and NF-Y are responsible for sterol-regulated transcription of the genes for human 3-hydroxy-3-methylglutaryl coenzyme A synthase and squalene synthase. *J Biochem* 123: 1191–1198
63 Naar AM, Beaurang PA, Robinson KM, Oliner JD, Avizonis D, Scheek S, Zwicker J, Kadonaga JT, Tjian R (1998) Chromatin, TAFs, and a novel multiprotein coactivator are required for synergistic activation by Sp1 and SREBP-1a *in vitro*. *Genes Dev* 12: 3020–3031
64 Natarajan R, Ghosh S, Grogan WM (1998) Molecular cloning of the promoter for rat hepatic neutral cholesterol ester hydrolase: evidence for transcriptional regulation by sterols. *Biochem Biophys Res Commun* 243: 349–355
65 Swinnen JV, Alen P, Heyns W, Verhoeven G (1998) Identification of diazepam-binding inhibitor/acyl-coA-binding protein as a sterol regulatory element-binding protein-responsive gene. *J Biol Chem* 273: 19938–19944
66 Bennett MK, Ngo TT, Athanikar JN, Rosenfeld JM, Osborne TF (1999) Co-stimulation of promoter for low density lipoprotein receptor gene by sterol regulatory element-binding protein and Sp1 is specifically disrupted by the yin yang 1 protein. *J Biol Chem* 274: 13025–13032
67 Ericsson J, Usheva A, Edwards PA (1999) YY1 is a negative regulator of transcription of three sterol regulatory element-binding protein-responsive genes. *J Biol Chem* 274: 14508–14513
68 Gauthier B, Robb M, Gaudet F, Ginsburg GS, McPherson R (1999) Characterization of a choles-

terol response element (CRE) in the promoter of the cholesteryl ester transfer protein gene: functional role of the transcription factors SREBP-1a, -2, and YY1. *J Lipid Res* 40: 1284–1293
69 Natarajan R, Ghosh S, Grogan WM (1999) Regulation of the rat neutral cytosolic cholesteryl ester hydrolase promoter by hormones and sterols: a role for nuclear factor-Y in the sterol-mediated response. *J Lipid Res* 40: 2091–2098
70 Bennett MK and Osborne TF (2000) Nutrient regulation of gene expression by the sterol regulatory element binding proteins: increased recruitment of gene-specific coregulatory factors and selective hyperacetylation of histone H3 *in vivo*. *Proc Natl Acad Sci USA* 97: 6340–6344
71 Xiong S, Chirala SS, Wakil SJ (2000) Sterol regulation of human fatty acid synthase promoter I requires nuclear factor-Y- and Sp-1-binding sites. *Proc Natl Acad Sci USA* 97: 3948–3953
72 Kim JH, Lee JN, Paik YK (2001) Cholesterol biosynthesis from lanosterol. a concerted role for sp1 and nf-y-binding sites for sterol-mediated regulation of rat 7-dehydrocholesterol reductase gene expression. *J Biol Chem* 276: 18153–18160
73 Shea-Eaton W, Lopez D, McLean MP (2001) Yin yang 1 protein negatively regulates high-density lipoprotein receptor gene transcription by disrupting binding of sterol regulatory element binding protein to the sterol regulatory element. *Endocrinology* 142: 49–58
74 Oliner JD, Andresen JM, Hansen SK, Zhou S, Tjian R (1996) SREBP transcriptional activity is mediated through an interaction with the CREB-binding protein. *Genes Dev* 10: 2903–2911
75 Ericsson J, Edwards PA (1998) CBP is required for sterol-regulated and sterol regulatory element-binding protein-regulated transcription. *J Biol Chem* 273: 17865–17870
76 Naar AM, Beaurang PA, Zhou S, Abraham S, Solomon W, Tjian R (1999) Composite co-activator ARC mediates chromatin-directed transcriptional activation. *Nature* 398: 828–832
77 Hua X, Sakai J, Ho YK, Goldstein JL, Brown MS (1995) Hairpin orientation of sterol regulatory element-binding protein-2 in cell membranes as determined by protease protection. *J Biol Chem* 270: 29422–29427
78 Brown MS, Goldstein JL (1999) A proteolytic pathway that controls the cholesterol content of membranes, cells, and blood. *Proc Natl Acad Sci USA* 96: 11041–11048
79 Sakai J, Nohturfft A, Goldstein JL, Brown MS (1998) Cleavage of sterol regulatory element-binding proteins (SREBPs) at site-1 requires interaction with SREBP cleavage-activating protein. Evidence from *in vivo* competition studies. *J Biol Chem* 273: 5785–5793
80 Duncan EA, Brown MS, Goldstein JL, Sakai J (1997) Cleavage site for sterol-regulated protease localized to a Leu-Ser bond in the lumenal loop of sterol regulatory element-binding protein-2. *J Biol Chem* 272: 12778–12785
81 Sakai J, Duncan EA, Rawson RB, Hua X, Brown MS, Goldstein JL (1996) Sterol-regulated release of SREBP-2 from cell membranes requires two sequential cleavages, one within a transmembrane segment. *Cell* 85: 1037–1046
82 Rawson RB, Zelenski NG, Nijhawan D, Ye J, Sakai J, Hasan MT, Chang TY, Brown MS, Goldstein JL (1997) Complementation cloning of S2P, a gene encoding a putative metalloprotease required for intramembrane cleavage of SREBPs. *Mol Cell* 1: 47–57
83 Duncan EA, Dave UP, Sakai J, Goldstein JL, Brown MS (1998) Second-site cleavage in sterol regulatory element-binding protein occurs at transmembrane junction as determined by cysteine panning. *J Biol Chem* 273: 17801–17809
84 Brown MS, Ye J, Rawson RB, Goldstein JL (2000) Regulated intramembrane proteolysis: a control mechanism conserved from bacteria to humans. *Cell* 100: 391–398
85 Hua X, Nohturfft A, Goldstein JL, Brown MS (1996) Sterol resistance in CHO cells traced to point mutation in SREBP cleavage-activating protein. *Cell* 87: 415–426
86 Hua X, Sakai J, Brown MS, Goldstein JL (1996) Regulated cleavage of sterol regulatory element binding proteins requires sequences on both sides of the endoplasmic reticulum membrane. *J Biol Chem* 271: 10379–10384
87 Rawson RB, DeBose-Boyd R, Goldstein JL, Brown MS (1999) Failure to cleave sterol regulatory element-binding proteins (SREBPs) causes cholesterol auxotrophy in Chinese hamster ovary cells with genetic absence of SREBP cleavage-activating protein. *J Biol Chem* 274: 28549–28556
88 Nohturfft A, Brown MS, Goldstein JL (1998) Topology of SREBP cleavage-activating protein, a polytopic membrane protein with a sterol-sensing domain. *J Biol Chem* 273: 17243–17250
89 Sakai J, Nohturfft A, Cheng D, Ho YK, Brown MS, Goldstein JL (1997) Identification of complexes between the COOH-terminal domains of sterol regulatory element-binding proteins (SREBPs) and SREBP cleavage-activating protein. *J Biol Chem* 272: 20213–20221
90 Nohturfft A, Hua X, Brown MS, Goldstein JL (1996) Recurrent G-to-A substitution in a single

codon of SREBP cleavage-activating protein causes sterol resistance in three mutant Chinese hamster ovary cell lines. *Proc Natl Acad Sci USA* 93: 13709–13714
91 Nohturfft A, Brown MS, Goldstein JL (1998) Sterols regulate processing of carbohydrate chains of wild-type SREBP cleavage-activating protein (SCAP), but not sterol-resistant mutants Y298C or D443N. *Proc Natl Acad Sci USA* 95: 12848–12853
92 Gil G, Faust JR, Chin DJ, Goldstein JL, Brown MS (1985) Membrane-bound domain of HMG CoA reductase is required for sterol-enhanced degradation of the enzyme. *Cell* 41: 249–258
93 Loftus SK, Morris JA, Carstea ED, Gu JZ, Cummings C, Brown A, Ellison J, Ohno K, Rosenfeld MA, Tagle DA et al (1997) Murine model of Niemann-Pick C disease: mutation in a cholesterol homeostasis gene. *Science* 277: 232–235
94 Nakajima A, Ohnishi S, Mimura T, Kubo K, Suzuki A, Yazaki Y, Matsuhashi N (2000) Protein-losing enteropathy associated with hypocomplementemia and anti-nuclear antibodies. *J Gastroenterol* 35: 627–630
95 Kumagai H, Chun KT, Simoni RD (1995) Molecular dissection of the role of the membrane domain in the regulated degradation of 3-hydroxy-3-methylglutaryl coenzyme A reductase. *J Biol Chem* 270: 19107–19113
96 DeBose-Boyd RA, Brown MS, Li WP, Nohturfft A, Goldstein JL, Espenshade PJ (1999) Transport-dependent proteolysis of SREBP: relocation of site-1 protease from Golgi to ER obviates the need for SREBP transport to Golgi. *Cell* 99: 703–712
97 Espenshade PJ, Cheng D, Goldstein JL, Brown MS (1999) Autocatalytic processing of site-1 protease removes propeptide and permits cleavage of sterol regulatory element-binding proteins. *J Biol Chem* 274: 22795–22804
98 Nohturfft A, DeBose-Boyd RA, Scheek S, Goldstein JL, Brown MS (1999) Sterols regulate cycling of SREBP cleavage-activating protein (SCAP) between endoplasmic reticulum and Golgi. *Proc Natl Acad Sci USA* 96: 11235–11240
99 Nohturfft A, Yabe D, Goldstein JL, Brown MS, Espenshade PJ (2000) Regulated step in cholesterol feedback localized to budding of SCAP from ER membranes. *Cell* 102: 315–323
100 Wang X, Pai JT, Wiedenfeld EA, Medina JC, Slaughter CA, Goldstein JL, Brown MS (1995) Purification of an interleukin-1 β converting enzyme-related cysteine protease that cleaves sterol regulatory element-binding proteins between the leucine zipper and transmembrane domains. *J Biol Chem* 270: 18044–18050
101 Tewari M, Quan LT, O'Rourke K, Desnoyers S, Zeng Z, Beidler DR, Poirier GG, Salvesen GS, Dixit VM (1995) Yama/CPP32 beta, a mammalian homolog of CED- is a CrmA-inhibitable protease that cleaves the death substrate poly(ADP-ribose) polymerase. *Cell* 81: 801–809
102 Nicholson DW, Ali A, Thornberry NA, Vaillancourt JP, Ding CK, Gallant M, Gareau Y, Griffin PR, Labelle M, Lazebnik YA (1995) Identification and inhibition of the ICE/CED-3 protease necessary for mammalian apoptosis. *Nature* 376: 37–43
103 Wang X, Zelenski NG, Yang J, Sakai J, Brown MS, Goldstein JL (1996) Cleavage of sterol regulatory element binding proteins (SREBPs) by CPP32 during apoptosis. *EMBO J* 15: 1012–1020
104 Pai JT, Brown MS, Goldstein JL (1996) Purification and cDNA cloning of a second apoptosis-related cysteine protease that cleaves and activates sterol regulatory element binding proteins. *Proc Natl Acad Sci USA* 93: 5437–5442
105 Nagoshi E, Imamoto N, Sato R, Yoneda Y (1999) Nuclear import of sterol regulatory element-binding protein- a basic helix-loop-helix-leucine zipper (bHLH-Zip)-containing transcription factor, occurs through the direct interaction of importin beta with HLH-Zip. *Mol Biol Cell* 10: 2221–2233
106 Nagoshi E, Yoneda Y (2001) Dimerization of sterol regulatory element-binding protein 2 via the helix-loop-helix-leucine zipper domain is a prerequisite for its nuclear localization mediated by importin beta. *Mol Cell Biol* 21: 2779–2789
107 Osborne TF, Gil G, Goldstein JL, Brown MS (1988) Operator constitutive mutation of 3-hydroxy-3-metylglutaryl-coenzyme A reductase promotor abolishes protein binding to sterol regulatory element. *J Biol Chem* 263: 3380–3387
108 Smith JR, Osborne TF, Brown MS, Goldstein JL, Gil G (1988) Multiple sterol regulatory elements in promotor for hamster 3-hydroxy-3-metylglutaryl-coenzyme A synthases. *J Biol Chem* 263: 18480–18487
109 Osborne TF (1991) Single nucleotide resolution of sterol regulatory region in promoter for 3-hydroxy-3-methylglutaryl coenzyme A reductase. *J Biol Chem* 266: 13947–13951
110 Sato R, Takano T (1995) Regulation of intracellular cholesterol metabolism. *Cell Struct Funct* 20:

421–427
111 Yang J, Sato R, Goldstein JL, Brown MS (1994) Sterol-resistant transcription in CHO cells caused by gene rearrangement that truncates SREBP-2. *Genes Dev* 8: 1910–1919
112 Kawabe Y, Sato R, Matsumoto A, Honda M, Wada Y, Yazaki Y, Endo A, Takano T, Itakura H, Kodama T (1996) Regulation of fatty acid synthase expression by cholesterol in human cultured cells. *Biochem Biophys Res Commun* 219: 515–520
113 Vallett SM, Sanchez HB, Rosenfeld JM, Osborne TF (1996) A direct role for sterol regulatory element binding protein in activation of 3-hydroxy-3-methylglutaryl coenzyme A reductase gene. *J Biol Chem* 271: 12247–12253
114 Bist A, Fielding PE, Fielding CJ (1997) Two sterol regulatory element-like sequences mediate up-regulation of caveolin gene transcription in response to low density lipoprotein-free cholesterol. *Proc Natl Acad Sci USA* 94: 10693–10698
115 Swinnen JV, Ulrix W, Heyns W, Verhoeven G (1997) Coordinate regulation of lipogenic gene expression by androgens: evidence for a cascade mechanism involving sterol regulatory element binding proteins. *Proc Natl Acad Sci USA* 94: 12975–12980
116 Sztrolovics R, Wang SP, Lapierre P, Chen HS, Robert MF, Mitchell GA (1997) Hormone-sensitive lipase (Lipe): sequence analysis of the 129Sv mouse Lipe gene. *Mamm Genome* 8: 86–89
117 Bruce C, Chouinard RA, Tall AR (1998) Plasma lipid transfer proteins, high-density lipoproteins, and reverse cholesterol transport. *Annu Rev Nutr* 18: 297–330
118 Chouinard RA Jr, Luo Y, Osborne TF, Walsh A, Tall AR (1998) Sterol regulatory element binding protein-1 activates the cholesteryl ester transfer protein Gene *in vivo* but is not required for sterol up-regulation of gene expression. *J Biol Chem* 273: 22409–22414
119 Guan G, Dai PH, Osborne TF, Kim JB, Shechter I (1997) Multiple sequence elements are involved in the transcriptional regulation of the human squalene synthase gene. *J Biol Chem* 272: 10295–10302
120 Kan HY, Pissios P, Chambaz J, Zannis VI (1999) DNA binding specificity and transactivation properties of SREBP-2 bound to multiple sites on the human apoA-II promoter. *Nucleic Acids Res* 27: 1104–1117
121 Pissios P, Kan HY, Nagaoka S, Zannis VI (1999) SREBP-1 binds to multiple sites and transactivates the human ApoA-II promoter *in vitro*: SREBP-1 mutants defective in DNA binding or transcriptional activation repress ApoA-II promoter activity. *Arterioscler Thromb Vasc Biol* 19: 1456–1469
122 Lopez D, McLean MP (1999) Sterol regulatory element-binding protein-1a binds to cis elements in the promoter of the rat high density lipoprotein receptor SR-BI gene. *Endocrinology* 140: 5669–5681
123 Foretz M, Pacot C, Dugail I, Lemarchand P, Guichard C, Le Liepvre X, Berthelier-Lubrano C, Spiegelman BM, Kim JB, Ferre P et al (1999) ADD1/SREBP-1c is required in the activation of hepatic lipogenic gene expression by glucose. *Mol Cell Biol* 19: 3760–3768
124 Foretz M, Guichard C, Ferre P, Foufelle F (1999) Sterol regulatory element binding protein-1c is a major mediator of insulin action on the hepatic expression of glucokinase and lipogenesis-related genes. *Proc Natl Acad Sci USA* 96: 12737–12742
125 Fra AM, Pasqualetto E, Mancini M, Sitia R (2000) Genomic organization and transcriptional analysis of the human genes coding for caveolin-1 and caveolin-2. *Gene* 243: 75–83
126 Incardona JP and Eaton S (2000) Cholesterol in signal transduction. *Curr Opin Cell Biol* 12: 193–203
127 Mater MK, Thelen AP, Pan DA, Jump DB (1999) Sterol response element-binding protein 1c (SREBP1c) is involved in the polyunsaturated fatty acid suppression of hepatic S14 gene transcription. *J Biol Chem* 274: 32725–32732
128 Bist A, Fielding CJ, Fielding PE (2000) p53 regulates caveolin gene transcription, cell cholesterol, and growth by a novel mechanism. *Biochemistry* 39: 1966–1972
129 Moon YA, Lee JJ, Park SW, Ahn YH, Kim KS (2000) The roles of sterol regulatory element-binding proteins in the transactivation of the rat ATP citrate-lyase promoter. *J Biol Chem* 275: 30280–30286
130 Sato R, Okamoto A, Inoue J, Miyamoto W, Sakai Y, Emoto N, Shimano H, Maeda M (2000) Transcriptional regulation of the ATP citrate-lyase gene by sterol regulatory element-binding proteins. *J Biol Chem* 275: 12497–12502
131 Schoonjans K, Gelman L, Haby C, Briggs M, Auwerx J (2000) Induction of LPL gene expression by sterols is mediated by a sterol regulatory element and is independent of the presence of

multiple E boxes. *J Mol Biol* 304: 323–334
132 Swinnen JV, Heemers H, Deboel L, Foufelle F, Heyns W, Verhoeven G (2000) Stimulation of tumor-associated fatty acid synthase expression by growth factor activation of the sterol regulatory element-binding protein pathway. *Oncogene* 19: 5173–5181
133 Frank PG, Galbiati F, Volonte D, Razani B, Cohen DE, Marcel YL, Lisanti MP (2001) Influence of caveolin-1 on cellular cholesterol efflux mediated by high-density lipoproteins. *Am J Physiol Cell* 280: C1204–1214
134 Lopez JM, Hegardt FG, Haro D (2001) Differential expression of cytosolic and mitochondrial 3-hydroxy-3-methylglutaryl CoA synthases during adipocyte differentiation. *Mol Cell Biochem* 217: 57–66
135 Shea-Eaton WK, Trinidad MJ, Lopez D, Nackley A, McLean MP (2001) Sterol regulatory element binding protein-1a regulation of the steroidogenic acute regulatory protein gene. *Endocrinology* 142: 1525–1533
136 Zannis VI, Kan HY, Kritis A, Zanni E, Kardassis D (2001) Transcriptional regulation of the human apolipoprotein genes. *Front Biosci* 6: D456–504
137 Rodriguez C, Martinez-Gonzalez J, Sanchez-Gomez S, Badimon L (2001) LDL downregulates CYP51 in porcine vascular endothelial cells and in the arterial wall through a sterol regulatory element binding protein-2-dependent mechanism. *Circ Res* 88: 268–274
138 Gondret F, Ferre P, Dugail I (2001) ADD-1/SREBP-1 is a major determinant of tissue differential lipogenic capacity in mammalian and avian species. *J Lipid Res* 42: 106–113
139 Christenson LK, Osborne TF, McAllister JM, Strauss JF 3rd (2001) Conditional response of the human steroidogenic acute regulatory protein gene promoter to sterol regulatory element binding protein-1a. *Endocrinology* 142: 28–36
140 Wang X, Sperkova Z, Napoli JL (2001) Analysis of mouse retinal dehydrogenase type 2 promoter and expression. *Genomics* 74: 245–250
141 Athanikar JN, Osborne TF (1998) Specificity in cholesterol regulation of gene expression by coevolution of sterol regulatory DNA element and its binding protein. *Proc Natl Acad Sci USA* 95: 4935–4940
142 Osborne TF (2000) Sterol regulatory element-binding proteins (SREBPs): key regulators of nutritional homeostasis and insulin action. *J Biol Chem* 275: 32379–32382
143 Sheng Z, Otani H, Brown MS, Goldstein JL (1995) Independent regulation of sterol regulatory element-binding proteins 1 and 2 in hamster liver. *Proc Natl Acad Sci USA* 92: 935–938
144 Shimano H, Horton JD, Hammer RE, Shimomura I, Brown MS, Goldstein JL (1996) Overproduction of cholesterol and fatty acids causes massive liver enlargement in transgenic mice expressing truncated SREBP-1a. *J Clin Invest* 98: 1575–1584
145 Horton JD, Bashmakov Y, Shimomura I, Shimano H (1998) Regulation of sterol regulatory element binding proteins in livers of fasted and refed mice. *Proc Natl Acad Sci USA* 95: 5987–5992
146 Horton JD, Shimomura I, Brown MS, Hammer RE, Goldstein JL, Shimano H (1998) Activation of cholesterol synthesis in preference to fatty acid synthesis in liver and adipose tissue of transgenic mice overproducing sterol regulatory element-binding protein-2. *J Clin Invest* 101: 2331–2339
147 Pai JT, Guryev O, Brown MS, Goldstein JL (1998) Differential stimulation of cholesterol and unsaturated fatty acid biosynthesis in cells expressing individual nuclear sterol regulatory element-binding proteins. *J Biol Chem* 273: 26138–26148
148 Horton JD, Shimano H, Hamilton RL, Brown MS, Goldstein JL (1999) Disruption of LDL receptor gene in transgenic SREBP-1a mice unmasks hyperlipidemia resulting from production of lipid-rich VLDL. *J Clin Invest* 103: 1067–1076
149 Shimomura I, Hammer RE, Richardson JA, Ikemoto S, Bashmakov Y, Goldstein JL, Brown MS (1998) Insulin resistance and diabetes mellitus in transgenic mice expressing nuclear SREBP-1c in adipose tissue: model for congenital generalized lipodystrophy. *Genes Dev* 12: 3182–3194
150 Shimano H, Shimomura I, Hammer RE, Herz J, Goldstein JL, Brown MS, Horton JD (1997) Elevated levels of SREBP-2 and cholesterol synthesis in livers of mice homozygous for a targeted disruption of the SREBP-1 gene. *J Clin Invest* 100: 2115–2124
151 Kim JB, Spiegelman BM (1996) ADD1/SREBP1 promotes adipocyte differentiation and gene expression linked to fatty acid metabolism. *Genes Dev* 10: 1096–1107
152 Kim JB, Sarraf P, Wright M, Yao KM, Mueller E, Solanes G, Lowell BB, Spiegelman BM (1998) Nutritional and insulin regulation of fatty acid synthetase and leptin gene expression through ADD1/SREBP1. *J Clin Invest* 101: 1–9

153 Rosen ED, Walkey CJ, Puigserver P, Spiegelman BM (2000) Transcriptional regulation of adipogenesis. *Genes Dev* 14: 1293–1307

154 Tontonoz P, Hu E, Spiegelman BM (1994) Stimulation of adipogenesis in fibroblasts by PPARγ2, a lipid-activated transcription factor. *Cell* 79: 1147–1156

155 Brun RP, Kim JB, Hu E, Altlok S, Spiegelman BM (1996) Adipocyte differentiation: A transcriptional regulatory cascade. *Curr Opin Cell Biol* 8: 862–832

156 Brun RP, Kim JB, Hu E, Spiegelman BM (1997) Peroxisome proliferator-activated receptor γ and the control of adipogenesis. *Curr Opin Lipidol* 8: 212–218

157 Spiegelman BM (1998) PPAR-gamma: adipogenic regulator and thiazolidinedione receptor. *Diabetes* 47: 507–514

158 Desvergne B, Wahli W (1999) Peroxisome proliferator-activated receptors: nuclear control of metabolism. *Endocr Rev* 20: 649–688

159 Kim JB, Wright HM, Wright M, Spiegelman BM (1998) ADD1/SREBP1 activates PPARγ through the production of endogenous ligand. *Proc Natl Acad Sci USA* 95: 4333–4337

160 Shimomura I, Hammer RE, Ikemoto S, Brown MS, Goldstein JL (1999) Leptin reverses insulin resistance and diabetes mellitus in mice with congenital lipodystrophy. *Nature* 401: 73–76

161 Lawrence RD (1946) Lipodystrophy and hepatomegaly with diabetes, lipaemia and other metabolic distrurbances. A case throwing new light on the action of insulin. *Lancet* 1: 724–731

162 Seip M, Trygstad O (1996) Generalized lipodystrophy, congenital and acquired (lipoatrophy). *Acta Paediatr Suppl* 413: 2–28

163 Matsuda M, Korn BS, Hammer RE, Moon Y-A, Komuro R, Horton JD, Goldstein JL, Brown MS, Shimomura I (2001) SREBP cleavage-activating protein (SCAP) is required for increased lipid synthesis in liver induced by cholesterol deprivation and insulin elevation. *Genes Dev* 15: 1206–1216

164 Streicher R, Kotzka J, Müller-Wieland D, Siemeister G, Munck M, Avci H, Krone W (1996) SREBP-1 mediates activation of the low density lipoprotein receptor promoter by insulin and insulin-like growth factor-I. *J Biol Chem* 271: 7128–7133

165 Shimomura I, Bashmakov Y, Shimano H, Horton JD, Goldstein JL (1997) Cholesterol feeding reduces nuclear forms of sterol regulatory element binding proteins in hamster liver. *Proc Natl Acad Sci USA* 98: 12354–12359

166 DeBose-Boyd RA, Ou J, Goldstein JL, Brown MS (2001) Espression of sterol regulatory element-binding protein 1c (SREBP-1c) mRNA in rat hepatoma cells requires endogenous LXR ligands. *Proc Natl Acad Sci USA* 98: 1477–1482

167 Repa JJ, Liang G, Ou J, Bashmakov Y, Lobaccaro JM, Shimomura I, Shan B, Brown MS, Goldstein JL, Mangelsdorf DJ (2000) Regulation of mouse sterol regulatory element-binding protein-1c gene (SREBP-1c) by oxysterol receptors, LXRalpha and LXRbeta. *Genes Dev* 14: 2819–2830

168 Yoshikawa T, Shimano H., Amemiya-Kudo M, Yahagi N, Hasty AH, Matsuzaka T, Okazaki H, Tamura Y, Iizuka Y, Ohashi K et al (2001) Identification of liver X receptor-retinoid X receptor as an activator of the sterol regulatory element-binding protein-1c gene promoter. *Mol Cell Biol* 21: 2991–3000

169 Ou J, Tu H, Shan B, Luk A, DeBose-Boyd RA (2001) Unsaturated fatty acids inhibit transcription of the sterol regulatory element-binding protein-1c (SREBP-1c) gene by antagonizing ligand-dependent activation of the LXR. *Proc Natl Acad Sci USA* 98: 6027–6032

170 Plutzky J (2000) Peroxisome proliferator-activated receptors in vascular biology and atherosclerosis: emerging insights for evolving paradigms. *Curr Ather Rep* 2: 327–335

171 Torra IP, Chinette G, Duval C, Furchart J-C, Staels B (2001) Peroxisome proliferator-activated receptors: from transcriptional control to clinical practice. *Curr Opin Lipidol* 12: 245–254

172 Martin G, Duez H, Blanquart C, Berezowski V, Poulain P, Fruchart J-C, Nauib-Fruchart J, Glineur C, Staels B (2001) Statin-induced inhibition of the Rho-signaling pathway activates PPARα and induces HDL apoA-I. *J Clin Invest* 107: 1423–1432

173 Dobbins RL, Szczepaniak LS, Bentley B, Esser V, Myhill J, McGarry JD (2001) Prolonged inhibition of muscle carnitine palmitoyltransferase-1 promotes intramyocellular lipid accumulation and insulin resistance in rats. *Diabetes* 50: 123–130

174 Unger RH, Zhou YT (2001) Lipotoxicity of β-cells in obesity and in other causes of fatty acid spillover. *Diabetes* 50 (Suppl. 1): S118-S121

175 Jacob S, Machann J, Rett K, Brechtel K, Volk A, Renn W, Maerker E, Matthaei S, Schick F, Claussen CD et al (1999) Association of increased intramyocellular lipid content with insulin

resistance in lean nondiabetic offspring of type 2 diabetic subjects. *Diabetes* 48: 1113–1119
176 Unger RH, Orci L (2001) Diseases of liporegulation: new perspective on obesity and related disorders. *FASEB J* 15: 312–321
177 Kakuma T, Lee Y, Higa M, Wang ZW, Pan W, Shimomura I, Unger RH (2000) Leptin, troglitazone, and the expression of sterol regulatory element binding proteins in liver and pancreatic islets. *Proc Natl Acad Sci USA* 97: 8536–8541

Cellular effects of HMG-CoA reductase inhibitors on blood cells (monocytes, macrophages, platelets)

Gerd Schmitz[1] and Michael Torzewski[2]

[1] *Institute for Clinical Chemistry and Laboratory Medicine, University Regensburg, Franz-Josef-Strauss-Allee 11, D-93053 Regensburg, Germany*
[2] *Johannes Gutenberg-Universität Mainz, Klinikum, Institut für Klinische Chemie und Laboratoriumsmedizin, D-55101 Mainz, Germany*

Atherosclerosis: an inflammatory disease

Atherosclerosis is the primary cause of ischaemic heart disease (IHD) and stroke and the leading cause of death and long-term disabilities in westernized societies. Several important environmental and genetic risk factors are associated with atherosclerosis. Over the past decade, it has become evident that atherosclerosis is not simply an inevitable degenerative consequence of ageing, but rather a chronic inflammatory condition connecting altered cholesterol metabolism and other risk factors to the development and progression of the atherosclerotic lesion and its sequelae like plaque rupture, fibrosis, calcification and thrombosis [1].

Eight histologically characteristic types of lesion were identified, and the Roman numerals with which they were designated give the usual sequence of lesion progression (Tab. 1). Lesion types I to IV are formed primarily through the accumulation of lipid in the intima. In types I and II, lipid accumulation occurs mainly intracellularly, in macrophages and smooth muscle cells (SMCs). Type III lesions contain, in addition, at least as much extracellular lipid. In type IV lesions, a confluent extracellular lipid core has been formed. In response to changes in the intima caused by the accumulated lipid alone, and more so if thrombotic deposits are present, intimal SMCs generate additional matrix, particularly collagen (type V lesions). Type VII is a lesion that is largely mineralized. The mineral (calcium) replaces earlier accumulation of lipid and dead cells. Similar lesions can be produced in animals by drastically reducing high serum cholesterol. Type VIII lesions consist mainly of layers of collagen, but they lack lipid. Such lesions also could be the result of lipid regression, or they could be the consequence of a thrombus that had formed in a part of the artery lacking lipid accumulation [2].

Cellular processes in atherogenesis are in principle not different from those in chronic inflammatory-fibroproliferative diseases such as liver cirrhosis, rheumatoid arthritis, glomerulosclerosis, pulmonary fibrosis, or chronic pan-

Table 1. Histological classification and terms used for atherosclerotic lesions

Type	Synonym	Effect on wall thickness and arterial lumen	Clinical correlation
Type I lesion	Initial lesions	no or minimal increase in wall thickness; no reduction in lumen	clinically silent
Type IIa lesion	Progression-prone type II		
Type IIb lesion	Progression-resistent type II		
Type III lesion	Preatheroma		
Type IV lesion	Atheroma	increased wall thickness but often only minimal lumen reduction	clinically overt or silent
Type V lesion	Fibroatheroma	additional increases in wall thickness; progressive reduction of the lumen	
Type VI lesion	Lesion with surface defect, hematoma-hemorrhage, and/or thrombotic deposit	thrombotic deposits increase lesion thickness; lumen often completely blocked	
Type VII lesion	Calcific lesion	wall thickened, lumen reduced	
Type VIII lesion	Fibrotic lesion		

creatitis. Atherosclerotic lesions are the result of a series of vessel-wall-specific cellular and molecular responses to various endogenous risk factors and potential exogenous antigens. These responses are mediated by endothelial cells, monocyte-derived macrophages, SMCs and specific subtypes of T-lymphocytes. Activation of these cells leads to the release of a wide spectrum of inflammatory hydrolases, cytokines, chemokines and growth factors, followed by cellular lipid accumulation and proliferation of SMCs, as well as formation of fibrous tissue. The modified response-to-injury hypothesis of atherosclerosis that emphasizes endothelial dysfunction, rather than denudation, as the first step in atherosclerosis was recently extended, suggesting that the key initiating event in early atherosclerosis is the subendothelial retention of cholesterol-rich, atherogenic lipoproteins bound to arterial proteoglycans (response-to-retention hypothesis) [3]. Following adherence to endothelial cells, defined subpopulations of circulating monocytes that express the lipopolysaccharide (LPS) receptor CD14 and the FcγRIII/CD16 are supposed to extravasate into the subendothelial space [4, 5]. Within the vessel wall, phagocytic monocytes rapidly transform into foam cells characterized by the excessive uptake of atherogenic lipoproteins (Tab. 2) via receptor-mediated endocytosis. Cellular uptake of these lipids and lipoproteins is mediated by charge and motif receptors (scavenger receptors) directly recognizing non-opsonized ligands [6]. Alternatively, modified lipids and lipoproteins may be opsonized by either

Table 2. Atherogenic lipids and lipoproteins

Lipids/lipoproteins	Atherogenic molecular component	Reference
oxidized LDL (ox-LDL)	hydroperoxy- and hydroxy fatty acids, secondary aldehydic lipid peroxidation products, 7 b-hydroperoxycholesterol	[119–121]
acetylated LDL (ac-LDL)	acetylated lipids	[122]
enzymatically degraded LDL (E-LDL)	free cholesterol, lysophospholipids	[123]
LDL-proteoglycan complexes	basic amino acid residues 3359–3369 in site B of apo-B100	[124]
lipoproteins aggregated by PLA2, PLC	lysophosphatidylcholine, phosphatidic acid, lysophosphatidic acid	[125, 126]
LDL hydrolyzed by sphingomyelinase	ceramide, phosphocholine	[127]
LDL hydrolyzed by phospholipase C	lysophosphatidylcholine, phosphatidic acid, lysophosphatidic acid	[128]
LDL modified by advanced glycation end products (AGEs)	67 amino acid domain located 1791 residues N-terminal to the LDL receptor binding site of apo-B	[129]
	modification of residues adjacent to the putative LDL receptor binding site	[130]
gangliosides (sialic acid containing glyco-sphingolipids)	sialic acid	[131]

innate non-specific opsonins (complement components, C-reactive protein (CRP), serum amyloid P (SAP), serum amyloid A_2 (SAA_2)) and/or specific opsonins (immunoglobulins) to facilitate cellular uptake mediated by different opsonin receptors including complement receptors, pentraxin family receptors and/or Fcγ receptors [6]. Continuous exposure to modified lipoproteins is supposed to trigger a chronic inflammatory process within the lesion. At the monocyte/macrophage level, this leads to the differentiation of either a phagocytic or an antigen-presenting phenotype with enhanced expression of procoagulant and pro-inflammatory genes as well as genes associated with lipid metabolism.

Controversy exists regarding the participation of innate immunity involving macrophages and natural killer (NK) cells *vs* antigen-specific acquired immunity involving lymphocytes. Macrophages predominate in atherosclerotic lesions. NK cells, although smaller in number, are present as well. T- and B-cells modulate disease progression and lesion development is reduced in mice lacking adaptive immunity. The presence of T-cells in addition to monocyte/macrophages in atherosclerotic lesions of both humans and animal models indicates that adaptive immunological events in conjunction with inflammatory ones are implicated in atherogenesis. T-lymphocytes, of both helper and suppressor phenotypes, have been identified within human atherosclerotic lesions displaying a shift during lesion progression [7]. Recent findings that dendritic cells (DCs) are present in the arterial wall and that their numbers increase in atherosclerotic lesions suggest that DCs could play a crucial role in T-cell activation in atherosclerosis [8]. Despite the predominance of T-cells, occasional B-cells were observed in advanced human atherosclerotic lesions [9]. Atherosclerosis is an inflammatory disease with a significant auto-immune component. Several auto-antigens and their respective auto-antibodies directed towards oxidized low-density lipoprotein (oxLDL), cardiolipin, β_2-glycoprotein-I and heat-shock protein 60/65, have been suggested as factors in human and murine atherogenesis [10]. Thus, innate immunity is necessary for atherosclerosis, whereas adaptive immunity is an important modulator of disease development [11, 12].

At the SMC level, complement activation by, e.g., CRP, SAA_2 or hydrolase-modified LDL takes place even in the early atherosclerotic lesions. Sublytic complement attack on SMCs leads to the local release of monocyte chemotactic protein 1 (MCP-1), a specific monocyte chemoattractant [13].

Monocytes/macrophages and dendritic cells in atheroclerosis

Cholesterol-loaded macrophages are critical components of atherosclerotic lesions and recent *in vivo* studies have demonstrated the importance of macrophages in lesion progression [14]. Vessel wall macrophages and antigen-presenting cells (APCs) form different lineages that originate from $CD34^+$ progenitor cells in the bone marrow [5].

The recent finding that in addition to phagocytic macrophages, increased numbers of DCs are found in atherosclerotic lesions [15] suggests that DCs, as the major classes of APCs, could play a crucial role in T-cell activation in atherosclerosis. Their current use in cancer immunotherapy, autoimmunity and transplantation combined with cellular vaccination [8] has made it possible to produce *in vitro* DCs with desirable properties to be therapeutically instrumental for the treatment of atherosclerosis.

In contrast to DCs, phagocytic macrophages are CD14/LPS receptor-positive and express high numbers of scavenger receptors and Fcγ receptors. Based on the current knowledge, the initially more restricted definition of scavenger receptors, i.e., as receptors for modified lipoproteins on phagocytic cells, may have to be extended to a more generalized view on receptors involved in scavenger function in host defence, inflammation and tissue remodelling [6]. This notion would include a wide spectrum of pattern recognition receptors that facilitate the clearance of chemically aberrant molecules and opsonized structures and, concomitantly, are involved in the modulation of adhesion, migration, differentiation and also host response processes [5].

Considerable evidence has accumulated demonstrating that integrins are in functional cooperation with these membrane receptors to coordinate monocyte adhesion, migration and differentiation to phagocytically active scavenger cells, which involves integrins as common transducers for a panel of integrin-linked specific receptors. This paradigm includes GPI-linked receptors (uPAR, LPS receptor CD14), as well as transmembrane receptors (LRP, SRAs, CD36), and it is likely that future studies will identify additional cooperative interactions [5]. As a first breakthrough, we were able to demonstrate that both LPS and ceramide induced a co-association of CD14, complement receptor 3 (CD11b/CD18), CD36 and decay-accelerating factor (CD55) [16]. Clustering of signaling and scavenging competent receptors may therefore provide an interesting mechanism by which different ligands induce distinct cellular processes in cardiovascular disease like cellular uptake of native and modified lipids and lipoproteins. In particular, modified lipids and lipoproteins like enzymatically degraded LDL (E-LDL) might be recognized via opsonin-mediated processes by either innate (complement components, CRP, SAP, SAA_2) and/or specific opsonins (immunoglobulins) prior to cellular uptake via opsonin receptors.

In human atherosclerosis, the most promising candidate for an innate opsonin at present is CRP, which has been classified as an innate recognition lectin [17]. During the last five years, the predictive association between the acute phase proteins CRP and Serum Amyloid A (SAA) and coronary heart disease (CHD) has been extensively confirmed [18, 19]. CRP is emerging as a key modulator of inflammatory processes already in early atherogenesis, in particular by its known complement-activating [20], lipoprotein-binding [21] and -opsonizing as well as chemotactic [22] properties. Of particular importance might be calcium-dependent *in vitro* binding of CRP to E-LDL accompanied by an enhancement of complement activation [23]. Different receptors have been described for CRP and, on monocytes, specific CRP binding occurs through FcγRI/CD64 [24] as well as FcγRII/CD32 [25].

Lineage and differentiation-dependent subsets of circulating blood monocytes and DC precursors express defined integrin patterns that parallel specific functional properties towards phagocytic capabilities or functions in antigen presentation, processes involved in foam cell formation and inflammatory reaction important for lesion progression in atherosclerosis. In normal subjects, 5 different subpopulations of blood monocytes were discriminated by cell expression densities of various antigens involved in extravasation, uptake of atherogenic lipoproteins, differentiation and inflammation. The Fcγ receptors, in particular CD16a/FcγRIII, together with the LPS receptor CD14, thereby turned out to be key surface markers for defining monocyte subpopulations. Their heterogeneous expression suggested a different capacity of IgG-dependent phagocytosis [26]. The pool size of CD14/CD16 monocytes (MNP 2 and MNP 3) correlates to plasma lipids and lipoprotein metabolism, as well as inflammation and the acute phase reaction, indicating a link between peripheral blood monocyte heterogeneity and cardiovascular risk factors (Fig. 1) [27].

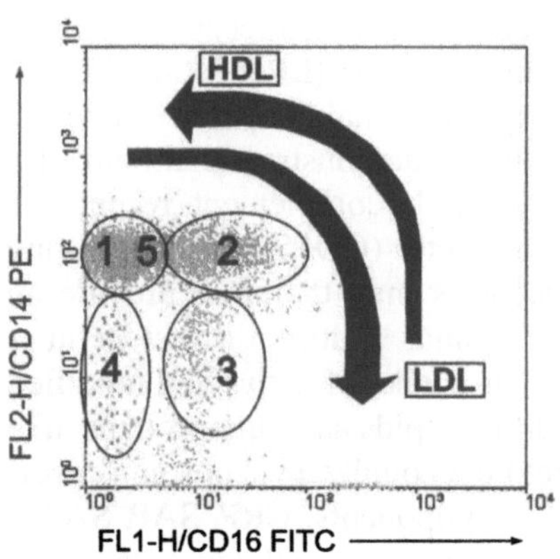

Phenotype of CD14^{dim}CD16^{+} Peripheral Blood Monocytes (MNP 3) Correlates

	Positively to	*Negatively to*	*Reference*
Plasma Lipids and Lipoproteins		HDL-cholesterol	[26]
	plasma cholesterol and triglycerides		[27]
	apoE4 allele		[4]
Inflammation, Acute Phase Reaction	M-CSF therapy		[113]
	GM-CSF therapy		[114]
	tuberculosis		[115]
	solid tumors		[116]
	sepsis		[33]
	HIV infection		[117, 118]

Figure 1. Correlation of the pool size of CD14^{dim}CD16^{+} monocytes (MNP 3) to plasma lipids and lipoprotein metabolism as well as inflammation and the acute phase reaction. Subpopulations of mononuclear phagocytes (MNP 1-5) were discriminated by flow-cytometry (left) due to their expression pattern of CD16a and CD14.

Pleiotropic effects of statins on monocytes and macrophages

Aside from their lipid-lowering activity, statins seem to possess relevant additional properties that target the phenotype of peripheral blood monocytes, platelet and endothelial dysfunction, leukocyte adhesion, macrophage stimulation, inflammatory and procoagulant responses and SMC transformation, as summarized in Table 3, to impair progression of atherosclerosis and to stabilize the atherosclerotic plaque [28, 29].

Effects on the phenotype of peripheral blood monocytes

Monocytes in peripheral blood are highly heterogeneous and specific functional changes are associated with their activation, differentiation and transformation to foam cells [26]. A subpopulation of 10% to 15% total monocytes is characterized by a phenotype similar to that of alveolar macrophages, as shown by expression of the FcγRIII/CD16 and only low expression of the LPSR/CD14 [30, 31]. After stimulation, this subset of macrophages similar to monocytes is capable of producing high levels of proinflammatory cytokines, such as tumor necrosis factor, in contrast to only low levels of the anti-inflammatory cytokine IL-10 [32]. The subset of CD14^{+}/CD16^{+} blood monocytes is expanded in sepsis patients, suggesting that septicemia may lead to substantial changes in blood monocyte composition [33]. Furthermore, increased expression of CD14 on monocytes throughout the acute phase of myocardial infarction has also been demonstrated [34].

In a previous study, it was demonstrated that low high-density lipoprotein (HDL)-cholesterol and the apo E4 allele are associated with an increased proportion of blood monocytes that are characterized by a high expression of

Table 3. *In vitro* pleiotropic effects of statins

Target	Stimulation	Inhibition	References
Endothelium	eNOS tPA uPA	PAI-1 Tissue factor Endothelin	[53, 132] [96, 133, 134] [135, 136]
Platelets		Adhesion Aggregation	[137]
Leukocytes			
Macrophages		MMP-9 secretion chemotaxis Tissue factor activity	[53, 96, 138]
NK cells		cytotoxicity	[139]
T-cells		cytotoxicity	[139]
SMCs	apoptosis TGF-β1	proliferation migration c-fos, c-jun PDGF ras and rho proteins ACE activity	[53, 134, 140] [141, 142]
osteoclasts		proliferation	[143]
fibroblasts, various tumor cells	apoptosis G1-arrest PI2-kinase inhibitor	S-phase progression	[144] [145, 146] [141, 147, 148] [149]

FcγRIII/CD16, a low expression of the LPS receptor (CD14) and a high expression of β_1- and β_2-integrins (Fig. 1). Recently, 79 hypercholesterolemic patients were treated either with the HMG-CoA reductase inhibitor fluvastatin in combination with diet or with placebo and diet in a double-blind and randomized multicenter study, and monitored for the potential effects on the phenotype of peripheral blood monocytes. At baseline, in the whole group of hypercholesterolemic patients, the population size of these more mature monocytes ($CD14^{low}CD16^{+}$) was positively correlated to triglyceride ($P = 0.003$) and total serum cholesterol levels ($P = 0.012$) [27]. Fluvastatin treatment for 52 weeks was associated with a 24.2% reduction in LDL-cholesterol ($P < 0.001$), as well as a 40.7% decrease in the expression density of CD14 on all monocytes ($P = 0.027$). A 24.5% decrease ($P < 0.001$) of the population of less differentiated $CD14^{high}CD16^{-}$ monocytes and an 83.1% increase ($P = 0.029$) of the population of more differentiated $CD14^{low}CD16^{+}$ monocytes further confirmed this modification of the phenotype of peripheral blood monocytes (Fig. 2). In conclusion, the positive pre-study correlation of the $CD14^{low}CD16^{+}$ monocyte subset to the serum cholesterol concentration, but inverse changes of both parameters under fluvastatin therapy indicate that

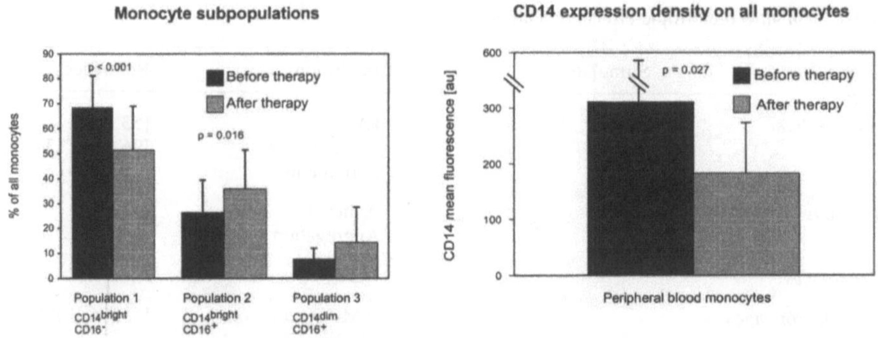

Figure 2. Phenotype of peripheral blood monocytes under inhibition of HMG-CoA reductase with fluvastatin.

fluvastatin exerts an as yet uncharacterized immunomodulatory effect on either monocyte maturation and differentiation, or extravasation which may also depend on the endothelial phenotype that is independent of the change in serum lipids. $CD14^{high}CD16^{+}$ monocytes (MNP 2) may be more reactive but $CD14^{low}CD16^{+}$ monocytes (MNP 3) may reflect a higher conversion rate of immature to differentiated monocytes or alternatively a shedding of CD14 from the surface as reported for stimulated monocytes [35]. In another recent study investigating the effect of simvastatin on monocyte adhesion molecule expression in patients with hypercholesterolemia, LDL levels correlated directly with both CD11b and CD14 expression and correlated inversely with L-selectin expression, showing that hypercholesterolemia affects monocyte adhesion molecule expression which, in turn, decreases with statin-induced plasmatic cholesterol reduction [36]. From these considerations two potential targets for statins are emerging: first, bone marrow progenitor cells leading to the maturation of less $CD14^{+}$ cells, and second, the blood compartment itself influencing differentiation and extravasation of monocytes.

Inhibition of cholesterol esterification and accumulation in macrophages

Studies performed in primary culture of mouse peritoneal macrophages (MPM) showed that fluvastatin may interfere with the esterification of cellular cholesterol elicited by acetylated low density lipoproteins (ac-LDL) [37]. Fluvastatin dose-dependently inhibited oleate incorporation into MPM cholesteryl esters. A similar result was achieved with simvastatin, but not pravastatin. Investigation of fluvastatin enantiomers showed the stereospecificity of drug action with most of the effects mediated by the (3R, 5S) antipode with the highest inhibitory activity on HMG-CoA reductase. Consistent with their effect on cholesterol esterification, fluvastatin and simvastatin reduced, in a concentration-dependent manner, the cellular content of esterified cholesterol by >70%. The reduction of cholesteryl esters induced by the drugs was not paralleled by a concomitant accumulation of cholesterol in its free form and led to a decrease of total cellular cholesterol [38]. Statins inhibit cholesteryl ester accumulation in monocyte-derived macrophages either by reducing the availability of free cholesterol towards the enzyme acyl-coenzyme A cholesterol acyltransferase by trapping it in phospholipid-containing pools, or by inhibiting LDL endocytosis related to reduced synthesis of mevalonate required for cholesterol esterification [37]. The addition of mevalonate or all-*trans* geranylgeraniol fully prevented the inhibitory effect of fluvastatin and simvastatin, suggesting that a non-sterol derivative(s) of mevalonate is involved in the endocytosis and esterification of exogenous cholesterol delivered to macrophages by modified LDL [38]. Besides cholesterol synthesis, the mevalonate pathway (Fig. 3) leads to the formation of dolichols, having an

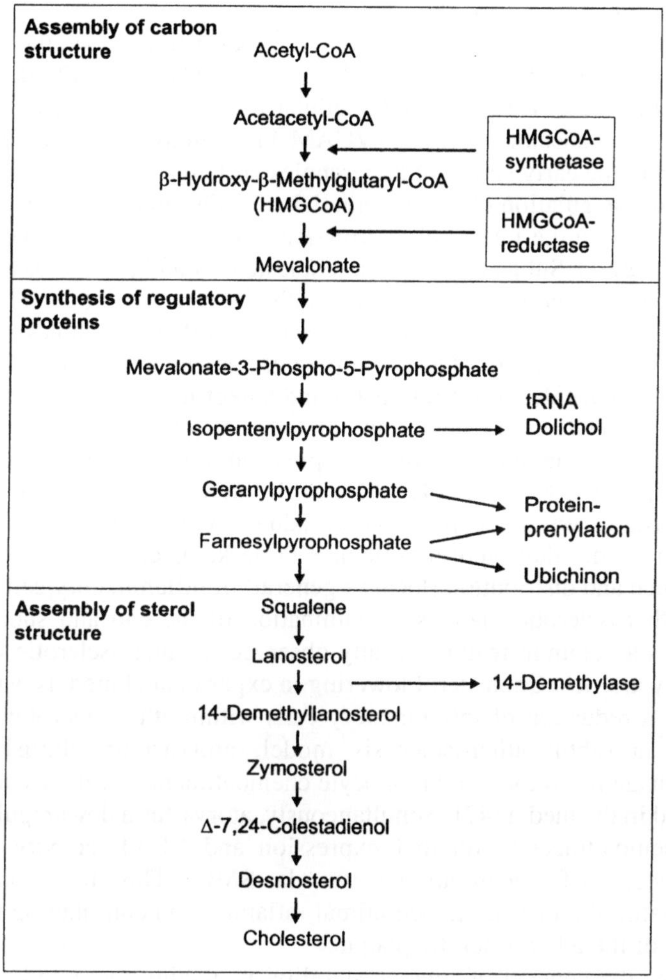

Figure 3. Cholesterol/mevalonate pathway.

essential role in lipoprotein synthesis, ubichinone, involved in electron transport, and isoprenoids, which take part in the farnesylation or geranylation of many proteins, including those needed for cell proliferation [39, 40]. Since virtually all cells possess the mevalonate pathway, it is not surprising that the influence of statins is not limited to the cardiovascular system.

Interestingly, data show that the efficacy of fluvastatin in inhibiting cholesterol esterification was greater in cholesterol-loaded than in normal cells, suggesting a possible specific and more pronounced effect on the atherosclerotic vessel wall. This might be due to the fact that, in cholesterol-rich cells, HMG-CoA reductase activity is already largely reduced as compared with unloaded cells [41].

Inflammation and plaque stability

An early step in atherogenesis involves monocyte adhesion to the endothelium and penetration into the subendothelial space. Scalia et al. [42] clearly demonstrated the role of P-selectin, intercellular adhesion molecule (ICAM-1), and vascular cell adhesion molecule (VCAM-1) in leukocyte-endothelium interaction during the early stages of hypercholesterolemia in the rabbit model. They observed upregulation of the endothelial cell adhesion molecules immunohistochemically in the intestinal microvascular endothelium of hypercholesterol diet-fed rabbits. Subjects with hypercholesterolemia have increased adhesiveness of isolated monocytes to fixed endothelial cells *in vitro*, and this response is diminished with lovastatin and simvastatin [43]. Hypercholesterolemic rats treated with fluvastatin have significantly attenuated leukocyte-adherence responses to platelet activation factor and leukotriene B_4 [44]. Indeed, cellular interaction between monocytes and endothelial cells was inhibited by fluvastatin, mediated via reduction of the expression of lymphocyte function-associated antigen-1 (LFA-1) and ICAM-1 [45]. Interestingly, the inhibitory effects of fluvastatin on the expression of adhesion molecules were completely reversed by the addition of mevalonate. Pasterkamp et al. [46] investigated the prevalence and distribution (local *vs* general) of inflammatory cells in nonruptured atherosclerotic plaques. Inflammation of the cap and shoulder of the plaque is a common feature, locally observed, in atherosclerotic femoral and coronary arteries. Cholesterol lowering in experimental models was accompanied by a reduction of inflammatory cells within atherosclerotic plaque [43, 44]. In a rabbit atherosclerosis model, atorvastatin abolished arterial macrophage infiltration and monocyte chemoattractant protein-1 in the neointima and in the media [47]. Simultaneously, atorvastatin downregulated monocyte chemoattractant protein-1 expression and NF-κB activity induced by tumor necrosis factor in cultured vascular SMCs. This study concluded that atorvastatin diminished the neointimal inflammation contributing to the stabilization of the atherosclerotic plaque.

Today, the concept of 'plaque stability' is gaining more and more importance. Plaque instability, manifesting as ulceration of the fibrous cap, plaque rupture and intraplaque hemorrhage, is characteristic of plaques with a high content of lipid and an excess of macrophages in the cap [48, 49]. Fibrous caps are often thin and macrophage-infiltrated at their shoulder regions, where disruption most frequently occurs [50]. Disrupted aortic caps contain fewer SMCs (the collagen-synthesizing cells) and less collagen than intact caps [48, 51]. Collagen is the main component of fibrous caps responsible for their tensile strength [51]. Macrophages are capable of degrading extracellular matrix by phagocytosis or by secreting proteolytic enzymes, in particular a family of metalloproteases (MMPs) that may weaken the fibrous cap, predisposing its rupture [52]. Lipids in the atheroma not only create mechanical instability, but also biologically active lipids participate in promoting oxidative stress and inflammatory responses such as monocyte migration. Lipid-lowering may therefore influence the matrix degradation cascade that appears most active in macrophage-rich areas of the atheroma, as well as promote mechanical stability within the plaque. Indeed, in addition to their effects on lipid accumulation in macrophages, statins have been recently shown to inhibit MMP production by macrophages in culture, an inhibition reverted by the addition of MVA [53], providing further insights on their direct anti-atherosclerotic potentials. In another study, Aikawa et al. [54] demonstrated that the lipid-lowering group showed progressive reduction in both macrophage content and matrix metalloproteinase-1 immunoreactivity with time. Aortic content of interstitial collagen increased in the lipid-lowering group compared with the baseline or continued hyperlipidemic group, indicating that lipid lowering reinforced the fibrous skeleton of the atheroma.

Effect of statin therapy on C-reactive protein levels

The predictive value of plasma CRP as a risk factor for cardiovascular events has led some researchers to support the use of CRP as a main cardiovascular risk assessment tool, along with total cholesterol: HDL ratios and homocysteine levels. The ability of HMG-CoA reductase inhibitors to lower CRP levels has recently brought into question the mechanisms of action of the statin drugs. Strandberg et al. [55] studied 60 hypercholesterolemic coronary patients who participated in the Treat to Target (3 T) study comparing atorvastatin and simvastatin. Serum lipids and CRP (with a sensitive method) were measured before treatment at baseline and after 12 months of statin treatment. LDL cholesterol was substantially decreased and HDL cholesterol increased during statin treatment. CRP decreased significantly (sign test $P = 0.03$) during treatment, and the changes of CRP were significantly associated with changes in HDL cholesterol ($r = -0.45$; $P < 0.001$) and apolipoprotein A1 ($r = -0.40$; $P < 0.001$) but not with changes in LDL cholesterol or triglycerides. The change in HDL cholesterol explained 20% of the change in CRP during statin treatment stressing the anti-inflammatory properties of HDL [55]. Very recently, the level of CRP was measured at baseline and after one year in 5742 participants in a five-year randomized trial of lovastatin for the primary prevention of acute coronary events. The results of this study suggested that statin therapy may be effective in the primary prevention of coronary events among persons with relatively low lipid levels but with elevated levels of CRP [56].

PRavastatin Inflammation CRP Evaluation (PRINCE) is an investigator-initiated, multicenter, community-based trial evaluating the effects of pravastatin on hs-CRP in up to 1182 individuals with coronary artery disease and up to 1702 individuals without coronary artery disease. Lipid profiles and hs-CRP levels were obtained at baseline, 12 weeks, and 24 weeks in all study participants. Patients with known coronary artery disease received 40 mg/d pravastatin, whereas those without coronary artery disease were randomly assigned to receive placebo or 40 mg/d pravastatin. In this prospective trial, pravastatin reduced CRP levels at both 12 and 24 weeks in a largely LDL-C-independent manner. These data provide evidence that statins may have anti-inflammatory effects in addition to lipid-lowering effects [57, 58].

Because statins lower incidences of acute cardiovascular events as well as decreasing morbidity and mortality well before the effects of lowered LDL cholesterol can be expected to occur, questions have been asked about whether they may work independently of LDL-lowering mechanisms.

T-lymphocytes in atherosclerosis

T-lymphocytes, of both helper and suppressor phenotypes, have been identified within human atherosclerotic lesions [59, 60] displaying a shift during lesion progression. In early atherosclerotic lesions, T-lymphocytes of suppressor phenotype appeared to predominate over helper cells. However, initial stages in the development of atherosclerosis also involve the infiltration of the arterial intima with Th1 cells reactive to heat shock protein (hsp) 65/60, expressed by endothelial cells in areas that are subject to increased hemodynamic stress [60] and Th1 cells responding to ox-LDL by proliferation and cytokine secretion [61]. In these early lesions, the ratio between T-cells and macrophages is approximately 1:8 [59]. In advanced atherosclerotic lesions, macrophages outnumber T-cells by 10 to 50:1 and $CD4^+$ T-cells are more than twice as frequent as $CD8^+$ cells. $CD4^+$ T-cells seem to be more important for acceleration of lesion formation, also due to the atherogenic role of the cytokine interferon-γ, which is produced by the Th1 subset of $CD4^+$ T-cells [62]. Thus, the cytokine expression in advanced human atherosclerotic plaques demonstrates the presence of a predominantly pro-inflammatory, Th1-type T-cell response [63]. Animal models, however, indicate that this cell type only modulates lesion development. Transgenic mouse models allow the conclusion that in the case of a lack of mature T-cells the development of fatty streaks is reduced under conditions of moderate hypercholesterolemia [64]. In contrast, in the case of extreme hypercholesterolemia, no protection against the development of atherosclerosis is observed in T- cell deficiency [65]. Taken together, these results indicate that in addition to the inflammatory cascade, a specific immune response mediated by T-cells may play a role in lesion progression, rather than lesion development [66].

Despite the predominance of T-cells, occasional B- and NK cells were observed in advanced human atherosclerotic lesions [65, 66]. Both early fatty streaks and full-blown atherosclerotic plaques of hypercholesterolemic apolipoprotein E knockout mice contained $CD22^+$ B-cells, suggesting that B-cells participate in the local immune response in this experimental model [68]. In addition, the detection of several auto-antigens and their respective auto-antibodies directed towards ox-LDL, cardiolipin, β_2-glycoprotein-I and heat-shock protein 60/65 stresses the importance of a humoral immune response in atherogenesis [10]. In aortic tissue, some of the infiltrating cells consist of NK cells and it was suggested that these cells may play a critical role in vascular cell injury and rupture caused by atherosclerotic aneurysms by releasing perforin [67].

Effects of statins on T-, B- and NK cell function

The attachment of monocytes and T-lymphocytes to the injured endothelium followed by their migration into the intima is one of the first and most crucial steps in lesion development. The co-localization of $CD4^+$ T-cells and macrophages in the lesion, the abundant expression of HLA Class II molecules and the co-stimulatory molecule CD40 and its ligand (CD40L) indicate a contribution of cell-mediated immunity to atherogenesis. Transgenic mouse models revealed that, depending on the model, T- and B-cells may promote lesion progression, whereas in contrast, monocytes and macrophages are essential for the development of atherosclerotic lesions [68].

T-cells are prominent components of both early and late atherosclerotic lesions and the role of Th1/Th2 cell subsets in the evolution and rupture of the plaque is currently under investigation. There are only a few reports dealing with the effects of statins on immune function. The results are controversial. Kwak et al. [69] showed that statins act as direct inhibitors of induction of MHC-II expression by IFN-γ and thus as repressors of MHC-II-mediated T-cell activation. This effect of statins was due to inhibition of the inducible promoter IV of the master regulator of MHC class II genes, CIITA (class II transactivator), and was observed in several cell types, including primary human endothelial cells and monocyte-derived macrophages. The inhibition was specific for inducible MHC-II expression and did not concern constitutive expression of CIITA and MHC-II. It was concluded that, in repressing induction of MHC-II, and subsequent T-lymphocyte activation, statins therefore provide a new type of immunomodulation. In line with these results, Arita et al. [70] showed that pravastatin treatment reduces nonspecific inflammation at the graft site and prevents early islet graft loss in a murine isograft model. The drug also inhibits neointimal proliferation in vascular allograft. These data were extended by demonstrating that statins (lovastatin and simvastatin) inhibit human T-cell interactions with elastin, a major protein of the adult vessel wall [71]. Upregulation of such interactions can be detected in vasculitis including atherosclerosis.

On the other hand, Montero et al. [72] investigated the effects of fluvastatin on Th1/Th2 cytokine release in relation to caspase-1 activation in human peripheral-blood mononuclear cells (PBMC) stimulated or not with *Mycobacterium tuberculosis*. Fluvastatin treatment resulted in the activation of caspase-1 and in secretion of interleukin (IL)-1β, IL-18, and IFN-γ (Th1). In the presence of bacteria, the release of these cytokines was highly increased by the statin in a synergistic way. By contrast, production of IL-12, IL-10 and IL-4 was unaffected by the statin. Not only did mevalonate abolish the effects of the statin but it also prevented the caspase-1 activation induced by the bacteria, suggesting the involvement of isoprenoids in the response to *M. tuberculosis*. The authors concluded that inhibition of HMG-CoA reductase may be immunoprotective by enhancing the Th1 response, which has therapeutical potential not only in atherosclerosis but also in infectious diseases.

The available data on the effects of HMG-CoA reductase inhibitors on NK cells and B-cells are controversial, too. Treatment of NK cells with compactin or lovastatin significantly abrogated the *in vitro* killing of a susceptible human erythroleukemic cell line. This inhibition was completely reversed by mevalonate [73]. Treatment with IL-2 also reversed lovastatin inhibition of NK cell function. In addition to natural cytotoxicity, IL-2 also restored chemotactic and antibody-dependent cellular cytotoxicity functions to lovastatin-treated cells. IL-2 had, however, no effect on the inhibition of cholesterol biosynthesis nor did it stimulate HMG-CoA reductase activity, supporting the hypothesis that there is a non-sterol isoprenoid product which is required for NK cell cytotoxicity and chemotaxis. In addition, the data suggested that IL-2 stimulation of NK cells proceeds by an isoprenoid-independent pathway [74]. McPherson et al. investigated the effect of lovastatin on a range of immune function parameters determined in a randomized, placebo-controlled, double-blind *ex vivo* study in 52 patients with primary hypercholesterolemia. No significant differences were found between lovastatin and placebo groups for basal NK or IL-2-induced cell-mediated cytotoxicity, PHA-stimulated lymphocyte proliferation, or relative numbers of T-lymphocytes ($CD3^+$), B-lymphocytes ($CD19^+$), total NK cells ($CD3^-$, $CD16^+$, $CD56^+$) and $CD57^+$ NK cells or in immunoglobulin levels after 4 or 8 weeks of treatment. Taken together, these inconclusive data point out the need for further studies on the effects of statins on NK and B-cell function.

Platelet activation

Experimental, clinical and epidemiological studies have demonstrated a unique role for platelets in the pathogenesis of atherothrombotic diseases, which have made obvious a great need for developing specific and effective drugs for the modulation of platelet function. Platelets circulate in the blood as non-adhesive, non-nucleated, disk-shaped cells, which upon activation undergo a series of discrete transformations. Platelet activation (Fig. 4), as a receptor-mediated response of resting platelets to specific stimuli, may be induced by subendothelial matrix proteins (e.g., von Willebrand factor (vWF), collagen) or specific soluble mediators such as thrombin, ADP, epinephrine or PAF. These receptor-mediated signaling processes trigger the reorganization of the cytoskeleton and the platelet shape change, as well as a redistribution of glycoproteins, the expression of a pro-coagulant surface, and the activation of the fibrinogen receptor GPIIb/IIIa [75]. Moreover, a degranulation of platelets results in the release of mediators such as ADP or serotonin, which further stimulate cellular activation, and growth factors such as PDGF, which may contribute to cellular proliferation, e.g., of vascular SMC. Platelet activation is a prerequisite for platelet aggregation, which finally results in the formation of a hemostatic plug as a natural response to injury. On the other hand, life-threatening occlusion of, e.g., coronary arteries upon plaque rupture causes mortality from atherosclerotic disease. Therefore, certain strategies have been pursued to modulate platelet function, which involve the inhibition of specific platelet agonists and the modulation of the intracellular cAMP/cGMP-system,

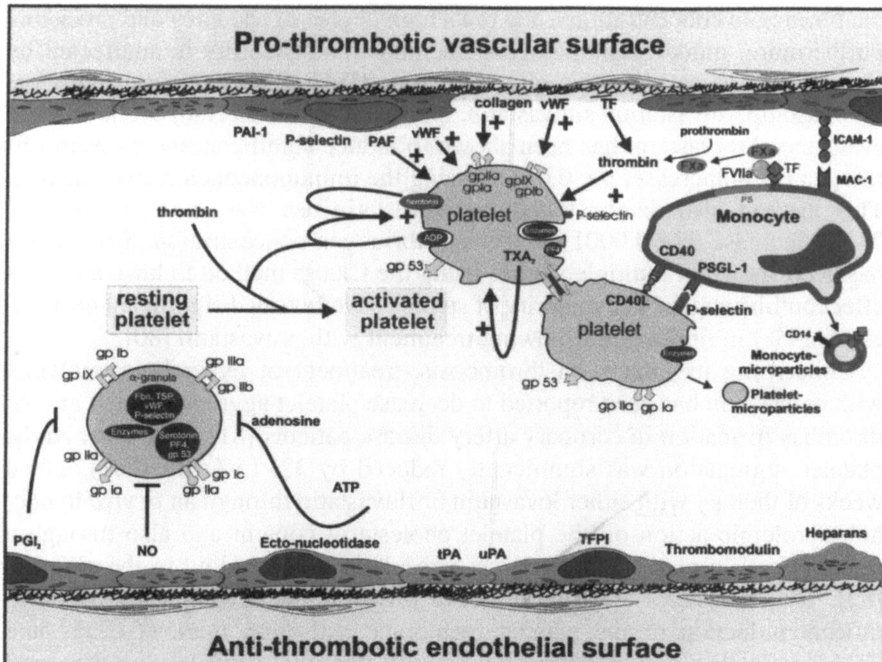

Figure 4. Mechanisms of platelet activation.

the antagonism of platelet aggregation via inhibition of fibrinogen binding and the inhibition of platelet thromboxane A_2 production.

Effects of statins on vascular hemostasis markers

Local activation of platelets and thrombus formation adjacent to atheromatous plaques, especially where ruptured or eroded, are recognized to be of pathophysiological importance in the acute and chronic clinical expression of CHD [76]. Favorable effects of statins on hemostasis may therefore be relevant to decreasing or delaying the progression and clinical manifestations of atherosclerosis. The hemostatic factors that have been evaluated with the statins include tissue factor (TF) and factor VII, thrombin generation, platelet aggregation, fibrinogen, plasma viscosity, and fibrinolytic factors.

Coagulation system

Platelets from patients with elevated LDL levels are more sensitive to aggregating agents than are platelets from normocholesterolemic subjects [77]. Hypercholesterolemia is associated with platelet activation in humans, detected as an increase in formation of thromboxane A_2, the principal prostaglandin generated by platelets and a potent platelet activator [78, 79].

The Clauss method is currently the preferred method for determining plasma fibrinogen concentrations, due to its high degree of accuracy and precision. Furthermore, unlike immunological methods, its reliability is unaffected by change in triglycerides. The effects of four HMG-CoA reductase inhibitors (atorvastatin, lovastatin, simvastatin, pravastatin) on fibrinogen have been evaluated. Atorvastatin has been shown to induce significant increases in fibrinogen (22% increase; $p < 0.05$) by using the immunonephelometric method. This method also demonstrated that lovastatin use was associated with a 24.4% increase ($p < 0.0001$) in plasma fibrinogen concentration. Simvastatin has been shown in multiple studies using the Clauss method to have a neutral effect on fibrinogen. The majority of studies have revealed significant decreases (7–19%) in fibrinogen following treatment with pravastatin [80].

Concerning its effects on thrombosis, treatment of hypercholesterolemia with pravastatin has been reported to decrease platelet aggregation and *ex vivo* thrombus formation in coronary artery disease patients [81]. In another study, platelet aggregation was significantly reduced by 12–15% ($p < 0.01$) after 4 weeks of therapy with either lovastatin or fluvastatin through an *in vivo* hypocholesterolemic action on the platelet cholesterol content and also through a direct effect on platelet function, as a result of drug binding to the platelets [82]. The cholesterol-lowering effect of fluvastatin is accompanied by a significant reduction of the platelet membrane activation markers CD62 and CD63, reflecting a reduced platelet activity that may contribute to the vasoprotective profile of fluvastatin [83]. Szczeklik et al. [84] determined the levels of prothrombin fragment 1+2 (F1+2) and FPA, thrombin cleavage products of prothrombin and fibrinogen, respectively, in hypercholesterolemic subjects. Simvastatin reduces platelet aggregation and thromboxane production after 4–24 weeks of therapy, whereas lipid lowering was observed by 2 weeks of treatment [79]. The generation of thrombin cleavage peptides in bleeding time blood was inhibited by simvastatin. Aspirin had a similar effect, and there was no further reduction in thrombin cleavage peptides by the addition of simvastatin to aspirin. A reduction in plasma levels of FPA or F1+2 could not be demonstrated. Dangas et al. [85] showed that plasma concentrations of FPA and F1+2 were unaffected by pravastatin in patients with hypercholesterolemia. However, pravastatin reduced thrombus generation in an *ex vivo* model where the patient's blood was passed through a perfusion system. The reduction in thrombosis was attenuated in patients on aspirin, again suggesting that aspirin and statins operate through the same pathway. These findings suggest that the reduction in thrombin generation by statins was secondary to an antiplatelet effect via specific inhibition of thromboxane A_2, the principal target of aspirin [86].

Lacoste and Lam have provided direct evidence for an antithrombotic effect of pravastatin and simvastatin in hypercholesterolemic coronary patients. There is also evidence that these patients have enhanced platelet aggregation. Treatment with simvastatin at a dose that reduced LDL-cholesterol by 30% to 40% in patients with hypercholesterolemia resulted in normalization of altered platelet aggregation *ex vivo* and a 50% reduction in thromboxane metabolite excretion when compared with placebo [79].

Thrombin is a potent stimulus of a wide variety of cells, including platelets, leukocytes, endothelial cells and SMCs, and can induce integrin expression, excretion, shape change, proliferation, angiogenesis and inflammation [87–90]. Such inductive processes involve the predominant thrombin receptor (proteinase-activated receptor-1 (PAR-1)) [91]. In response to thrombin stimulation (e.g., through PAR-1), cells express integrins (e.g., GMP-140) and other proteins (e.g., TF, factor VIIa, factor Xa and PAR-1) and secrete a variety of proteins (e.g., factor VIII and vWF). Statins are inhibitors of HMG-CoA reductase, which produces mevalonic acid at the third step in the isoprenoid pathways (Fig. 3). These pathways have four major branches, of which three produce cell-regulating substances and the fourth leads to cholesterol [92]. Thrombin is known to stimulate platelets and other cells through PAR-1 by G-protein-coupled mechanisms and upregulates proteins and kinases of the *ras* system, which are isoprenoid dependent [92, 93]. In a recent clinical study, the statin simvastatin at 20 mg daily was found to reduce in 2 months total cholesterol by 24%, prothrombin (FII) activation fragment by 35%, and monocyte TF activity and antigen by 61 and 68%, respectively [94]. Because TF participates in FII activation, thrombin is clearly implicated.

Brand et al. [95] demonstrated that oxLDL enhanced LPS-induced TF expression in human adherent monocytes. In this regard, lipophilic statins (fluvastatin, simvastatin) suppress TF expression by cultured human macrophages through inhibition of a geranylgeranylated protein involved in TF biosynthesis

[96]. Cerivastatin treatment also reduced TF expression in cultured human monocyte/macrophages [97]. This effect on TF was not observed with pravastatin. Ferro et al. [94] reported that simvastatin reduced monocyte TF expression in 24 patients with type IIa hypercholesterolemia, consistent with recent experimental data demonstrating that protein expression of TF diminished substantially in the rabbit low cholesterol group [98]. *In situ* binding of TF, factors VIIa and X colocalized with TF protein in atheroma and decreased after lipid lowering. Furthermore, TF biological activity was reduced in the low cholesterol group as determined by a chromogenic assay [98]. Therefore, this effect of statins may be mediated by lowering cholesterol, including LDL and/or by antioxidant effects [99].

Lovastatin and pravastatin have been shown to reduce cytosolic calcium and platelet aggregation [100]. Statins may reduce platelet aggregation by changing the cholesterol content of platelet membranes, which alters membrane fluidity [100]. On the other hand, Thomas and Mann [101] reported a significant increase in the frequency of thrombotic events after change of simvastatin to fluvastatin, suggesting that less potent statins and/or consequent increase in lipid may act to unleash an otherwise quiescent atheroma, with plaque instability leading to an increase in vascular events. Of interest is that atorvastatin and simvastatin resulted in severe thrombocytopenia in hypercholesterolemic patients, suggesting immune thrombocytopenia [102, 103].

Fibrinolysis system

Fibrinolytic mechanisms evaluated with statins include measurements of PAI-1, the principal inhibitor of the fibrinolytic system and lipoprotein(a). Gemfibrozil and pravastatin reduced PAI-1 plasma levels in hypercholesterolemic subjects [104, 105]. Recently, Bourcier and Libby [106] demonstrated that simvastatin reduced levels of PAI-1 antigen released from SMCs and endothelial cells. Levels of endothelial cell-derived tPA increased 2-fold over the same concentrations of simvastatin that inhibited release of PAI-1. Simvastatin's inhibitory effect was prevented by geranylgeranyl pyrophosphate, but not by farnesyl pyrophosphate, suggesting the involvement of geranylgeranyl-modified intermediates. Decreased PAI-1 antigen was correlated with reduced mRNA transcription and activity of the PAI-1 promoter [107].

Lovastatin administration has produced contradictory results in humans: with decreased PAI-1 antigen by 22% in one study [107] and elevated PAI-1 by 34% in another [108]. Pravastatin reduced PAI-1 antigen levels by 26–56% [109]. Simvastatin increased PAI-1 antigen by 18% in 111 patients treated for 2 years [110]. Fluvastatin had no effect on PAI-1 antigen [111]. Atorvastatin therapy increased PAI-1 antigen by 36% after 12 months [108]. In a recent study, simvastatin did not significantly change PAI-1 antigen levels from the pretreatment mean of 19.2–18.6 ng/ml in hypercholesterolemic postmenopausal women [112]. Furthermore, simvastatin did not significantly change serum D-dimer levels, cross-linked degradation products of fibrin. Thus, the effects of statins on fibrinolysis in humans remain unclear.

Conclusion

Independent of their ability to reduce plasma cholesterol, three potential targets for statins are emerging concerning leukocyte differentiation (Fig. 5): first, bone marrow progenitor cells, leading to the maturation of less $CD14^+$ cells, second, the blood compartment itself, influencing differentiation and extravasation of monocytes, and third, statins are able to reduce the *in vitro* cholesterol accumulation in macrophages (either directly or via reduction of plasma levels of potential opsonins like CRP) and expression of matrix metalloproteinases, resulting in plaque stability. Repressing induction of MHC-II, and subsequent T-lymphocyte activation, statins further provide a new type of immunomodulation. These activities, which affect major processes involved in the formation of atherosclerotic lesions, are linked to the local modulation of the mevalonate pathway. Accordingly, statins exert their cardiovascular benefits through direct anti-atherogenic properties in the arterial wall, beyond their effects on plasma lipids. Following plaque disruption, statins may influence thrombosis through variable inhibitory action on platelet deposition and aggregation, coagulation factors, thrombin generation, rheology and fibrinolysis. These effects of statins may contribute to the primary or secondary prevention of CHD in large clinical studies. However, the clinical significance of diverse effects of statins on factor VII, fibrinogen, plasma viscosity, PAI-1 and lipoprotein(a) has been not yet determined. Accordingly, understanding the effects of statins on hemostasis with respect to prevention or treatment of atherosclerosis will require further basic and clinical research.

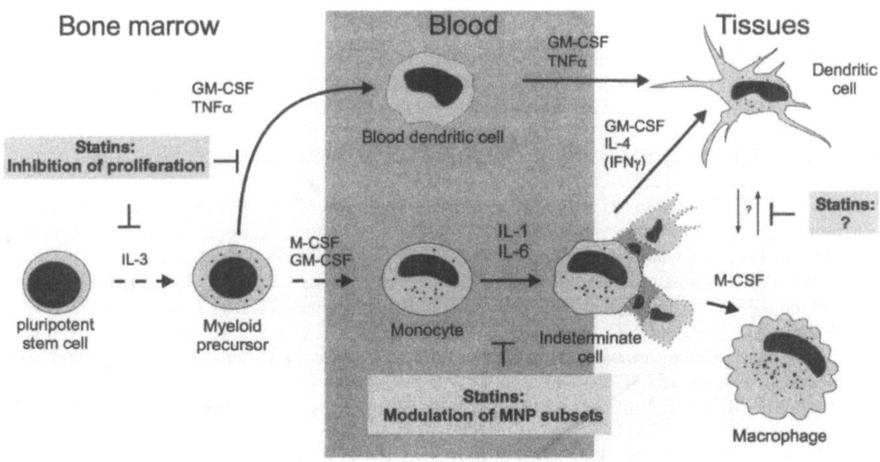

Figure 5. Potential targets for cholesterol synthesis blockers in monocyte differentiation.

References

1 Lusis A (2000) Atherosclerosis. *Nature* 407: 233–241

2 Stary HC (2000) Natural history and histological classification of atherosclerotic lesions: an update. *Arterioscler Thromb Vasc Biol* 20: 1177–1178

3 Williams KJ, Tabas I: (1998) The response-to-retention hypothesis of atherogenesis reinforced. *Curr Opin Lipidol* 9: 471–474

4 Stohr J, Schindler G, Rothe G, Schmitz G (1998) Enhanced upregulation of the Fc gamma receptor IIIa (CD16a) during *in vitro* differentiation of ApoE4/4 monocytes. *Arterioscler Thromb Vasc Biol* 18: 1424–1432

5 Schmitz G, Orso E, Rothe G, Klucken J (1997) Scavenging, signaling and adhesion coupling in macrophages: implications for atherogenesis. *Curr Opin Lipidol* 8: 287–300

6 Schmitz G, Torzewski M (2001) Atherosclerosis: An inflammatory disease. *In*: JL Metha (ed): *Inflammatory and Infectious Basis of Atherosclerosis*. Birkhäuser Verlag, Basel, 1–21

7 Hansson GK, Zhou X, Tornquist E, Paulsson G (2000) The role of adaptive immunity in atherosclerosis. *Ann N Y Acad Sci* 902: 53–62

8 Bobryshev YV (2000) Dendritic cells and their involvement in atherosclerosis. *Curr Opin Lipidol* 11: 511–517

9 Grewal IS, Flavell RA (1998) CD40 and CD154 in cell-mediated immunity. *Annu Rev Immunol* 16: 11–135

10 Shoenfeld Y, Sherer Y, George J, Harats D (2000) Autoantibodies associated with atherosclerosis. *Ann Med* 32 Suppl 1: 37–40

11 Hansson GK (1999) Inflammation and immune response in atherosclerosis. *Curr Atheroscler Rep* 1: 150–155

12 Curtiss LK, Kubo N, Schiller NK, Boisvert WA (2000) Participation of innate and acquired immunity in atherosclerosis. *Immunol Res* 21: 167–176

13 Torzewski J, Oldroyd R, Lachmann P, Fitzsimmons C, Proudfoot D, Bowyer D (1996) Complement-induced release of monocyte chemotactic protein-1 from human smooth muscle cells. A possible initiating event in atherosclerotic lesion formation. *Arterioscler Thromb Vasc Biol* 16: 673–677

14 Smith JD, Trogan E, Ginsberg M, Grigaux C, Tian J, Miyata M (1995) Decreased atherosclerosis in mice deficient in both macrophage colony-stimulating factor (op) and apolipoprotein. E. *Proc Natl Acad Sci USA* 92: 8264–8268

15 Bobryshev YV, Lord RS (1995) Ultrastructural recognition of cells with dendritic cell morphology in human aortic intima. Contacting interactions of vascular dendritic cells in athero-resistant and athero-prone areas of the normal aorta. *Arch Histol Cytol* 58: 307–322

16 Pfeiffer A, Böttcher A, Orso E, Kapinski M, Nagy P., Bodnar A, Speitzer I, Liebisch G, Drobnik W, Gempel K et al (2001) LPS and ceramide docking to CD14 provokes differential raft domain clustering. *Eur J Immunol* 31: 3153–3164

17 Fearon DT, Locksley RM (1996) The instructive role of innate immunity in the acquired immune response. *Science* 272: 50–53

18 Haverkate F, Thompson SG, Pyke SD, Gallimore JR, Pepys MB (1997) Production of C-reactive protein and risk of coronary events in stable and unstable angina. European Concerted Action on Thrombosis and Disabilities Angina Pectoris Study Group. *Lancet* 349: 462–466

19 Ridker PM, Cushman M, Stampfer MJ, Tracy RP, Hennekens CH (1997) Inflammation, aspirin, and the risk of cardiovascular disease in apparently healthy men. *N Engl J Med* 336: 973–979

20 Wolbink GJ, Brouwer MC, Buysmann S, Ten BI, Hack CE (1996) CRP-mediated activation of complement *in vivo*: assessment by measuring circulating complement-C-reactive protein complexes. *J Immunol* 157: 473–479

21 Pepys MB, Rowe IF, Baltz ML (1985) C-reactive protein: binding to lipids and lipoproteins. *Int Rev Exp Pathol* 27: 83–111

22 Whisler RL, Proctor VK, Downs EC, Mortensen RF (1986) Modulation of human monocyte chemotaxis and procoagulant activity by human C-reactive protein (CRP). *Lymphokine Res* 5: 223–228

23 Bhakdi S, Torzewski M, Klouche M, Hemmes M (1999) Complement and atherogenesis: binding of CRP to degraded, nonoxidized LDL enhances complement activation. *Arterioscler Thromb Vasc Biol* 19: 2348–2354

24 Marnell LL, Mold C, Volzer MA, Burlingame RW, Du CT (1995) C-reactive protein binds to Fc

gamma RI in transfected COS cells. *J Immunol* 155: 2185–2193
25 Bharadwaj D, Stein MP, Volzer M, Mold C, Du CT (1999) The major receptor for C-reactive protein on leukocytes is fcgamma receptor II. *J Exp Med* 190: 585–590
26 Rothe G, Gabriel H, Kovacs E, Klucken J, Stohr J, Kindermann W, Schmitz G (1996) Peripheral blood mononuclear phagocyte subpopulations as cellular markers in hypercholesterolemia. *Arterioscler Thromb Vasc Biol* 16: 1437–1447
27 Rothe G, Herr AS, Stohr J, Abletshauser C, Weidinger G, Schmitz G (1999) A more mature phenotype of blood mononuclear phagocytes is induced by fluvastatin treatment in hypercholesterolemic patients with coronary heart disease. *Atherosclerosis* 144: 251–261
28 Libby P, Aikawa M (1998) New insights into plaque stabilisation by lipid lowering. *Drugs* 56 Suppl 1: 9–13
29 Newby AC, Libby P, van der Wal AC (1999) Plaque instability-the real challenge for atherosclerosis research in the next decade? *Cardiovasc Res* 41: 321–322
30 Passlick B, Flieger D, Ziegler-Heitbrock HW (1989) Identification and characterization of a novel monocyte subpopulation in human peripheral blood. *Blood* 74: 2527–2534
31 Ziegler-Heitbrock HW, Fingerle G, Strobel M, Schraut W, Stelter F, Schutt C, Passlick B, Pforte A (1993) The novel subset of $CD14^+/CD16^+$ blood monocytes exhibits features of tissue macrophages. *Eur J Immunol* 23: 2053–2058
32 Frankenberger M, Sternsdorf T, Pechumer H, Pforte A, Ziegler-Heitbrock HW (1996) Differential cytokine expression in human blood monocyte subpopulations: a polymerase chain reaction analysis. *Blood* 87: 373–377
33 Fingerle G, Pforte A, Passlick B, Blumenstein M, Strobel M, Ziegler-Heitbrock HW (1993) The novel subset of $CD14^+/CD16^+$ blood monocytes is expanded in sepsis patients. *Blood* 82: 3170–3176
34 Meisel SR, Shapiro H, Radnay J, Neuman Y, Khaskia AR, Gruener N, Pauzner H, David D (1998) Increased expression of neutrophil and monocyte adhesion molecules LFA-1 and Mac-1 and their ligand ICAM-1 and VLA-4 throughout the acute phase of myocardial infarction: possible implications for leukocyte aggregation and microvascular plugging. *J Am Coll Cardiol* 31: 120–125
35 Bazil V, Strominger JL (1991) Shedding as a mechanism of down-modulation of CD14 on stimulated human monocytes. *J Immunol* 147: 1567–1574
36 Serrano CV, Yoshida VM, Venturinelli ML, D'Amico E, Monteiro HP, Ramires JA, da Luz PL (2001) Effect of simvastatin on monocyte adhesion molecule expression in patients with hypercholesterolemia. *Atherosclerosis* 157: 505–512
37 Bernini F, Didoni G, Bonfadini G, Bellosta S, Fumagalli R (1993) Requirement for mevalonate in acetylated LDL induction of cholesterol esterification in macrophages. *Atherosclerosis* 104: 19–26
38 Raiteri M, Arnaboldi L, McGeady P, Gelb MH, Verri D, Tagliabue C, Quarato P, Ferraboschi P, Santaniello E, Paoletti R et al (1997) Pharmacological control of the mevalonate pathway: effect on arterial smooth muscle cell proliferation. *J Pharmacol Exp Ther* 281: 1144–1153
39 Corsini A, Bellosta S, Baetta R, Fumagalli R, Paoletti R, Bernini F (1999) New insights into the pharmacodynamic and pharmacokinetic properties of statins. *Pharmacol Ther* 84: 413–428
40 Corsini A, Bernini F, Quarato P, Donetti E, Bellosta S, Fumagalli R, Paoletti R, Soma VM (1996) Non-lipid-related effects of 3-hydroxy-3-methylglutaryl coenzyme A reductase inhibitors. *Cardiology* 87: 458–468
41 Bernini F, Scurati N, Bonfadini G, Fumagalli R (1995) HMG-CoA reductase inhibitors reduce acetyl LDL endocytosis in mouse peritoneal macrophages. *Arterioscler Thromb Vasc Biol* 15: 1352–1358
42 Scalia R, Appel JZ, Lefer AM (1998) Leukocyte-endothelium interaction during the early stages of hypercholesterolemia in the rabbit: role of P-selectin, ICAM-1, and VCAM-1. *Arterioscler Thromb Vasc Biol* 18: 1093–1100
43 Weber C, Erl W, Weber KS, Weber PC (1997) HMG-CoA reductase inhibitors decrease CD11b expression and CD11b-dependent adhesion of monocytes to endothelium and reduce increased adhesiveness of monocytes isolated from patients with hypercholesterolemia. *J Am Coll Cardiol* 30: 1212–1217
44 Kimura M, Kurose I, Russell J, Granger DN (1997) Effects of fluvastatin on leukocyte-endothelial cell adhesion in hypercholesterolemic rats. *Arterioscler Thromb Vasc Biol* 17: 1521–1526
45 Niwa S, Totsuka T, Hayashi S (1996) Inhibitory effect of fluvastatin, an HMG-CoA reductase

inhibitor, on the expression of adhesion molecules on human monocyte cell line. *Int J Immunopharmacol* 18: 669–675
46 Pasterkamp G, Schoneveld AH, van der Wal AC, Hijnen DJ, van Wolveren WJ, Plomp S, Teepen HL, Borst C (1999) Inflammation of the atherosclerotic cap and shoulder of the plaque is a common and locally observed feature in unruptured plaques of femoral and coronary arteries. *Arterioscler Thromb Vasc Biol* 19: 54–58
47 Bustos C, Hernandez-Presa MA, Ortego M, Tunon J, Ortega L, Perez F, Diaz C, Hernandez G, Egido J (1998) HMG-CoA reductase inhibition by atorvastatin reduces neointimal inflammation in a rabbit model of atherosclerosis. *J Am Coll Cardiol* 32: 2057–2064
48 Davies MJ, Richardson PD, Woolf N, Katz DR, Mann J (1993) Risk of thrombosis in human atherosclerotic plaques: role of extracellular lipid, macrophage, and smooth muscle cell content. *Br Heart J* 69: 377–381
49 Fernandez-Ortiz A, Badimon JJ, Falk E, Fuster V, Meyer B, Mailhac A, Weng D, Shah PK, Badimon L (1994) Characterization of the relative thrombogenicity of atherosclerotic plaque components: implications for consequences of plaque rupture. *J Am Coll Cardiol* 23: 1562–1569
50 Richardson PD, Davies MJ, Born GV (1989) Influence of plaque configuration and stress distribution on fissuring of coronary atherosclerotic plaques. *Lancet* 2: 941–944
51 Burleigh MC, Briggs AD, Lendon CL, Davies MJ, Born GV, Richardson PD (1992) Collagen types I and III, collagen content, GAGs and mechanical strength of human atherosclerotic plaque caps: span-wise variations. *Atherosclerosis* 96: 71–81
52 Dollery CM, McEwan JR, Henney AM (1995) Matrix metalloproteinases and cardiovascular disease. *Circ Res* 77: 863–868
53 Bellosta S, Via D, Canavesi M, Pfister P, Fumagalli R, Paoletti R, Bernini F (1998) HMG-CoA reductase inhibitors reduce MMP-9 secretion by macrophages. *Arterioscler Thromb Vasc Biol* 18: 1671–1678
54 Aikawa M, Rabkin E, Okada Y, Voglic SJ, Clinton SK, Brinckerhoff CE, Sukhova GK, Libby P (1998) Lipid lowering by diet reduces matrix metalloproteinase activity and increases collagen content of rabbit atheroma: a potential mechanism of lesion stabilization. *Circulation* 97: 2433–2444
55 Strandberg TE, Vanhanen H, Tikkanen MJ (2000) Associations between change in C-reactive protein and serum lipids during statin treatment. *Ann Med* 32: 579–583
56 Ridker PM, Rifai N, Clearfield M, Downs JR, Weis SE, Miles JS, Gotto AMJ (2001) Measurement of C-reactive protein for the targeting of statin therapy in the primary prevention of acute coronary events. *N Engl J Med* 344: 1959–1965
57 Albert MA, Danielson E, Rifai N, Ridker PM (2001) Effect of statin therapy on C-reactive protein levels: the pravastatin inflammation/CRP evaluation (PRINCE): a randomized trial and cohort study. *JAMA* 286: 64–70
58 Albert MA, Staggers J, Chew P, Ridker PM (2001) The pravastatin inflammation CRP evaluation (PRINCE): rationale and design. *Am Heart J* 141: 893–898
59 Munro JM, van der Walt JD, Munro CS, Chalmers JA, Cox EL (1987) An immunohistochemical analysis of human aortic fatty streaks. *Hum Pathol* 18: 375–380
60 Wick G, Kleindienst R, Schett G, Amberger A, Xu Q (1995) Role of heat shock protein 65/60 in the pathogenesis of atherosclerosis. *Int Arch Allergy Immunol* 107: 130–131
61 Stemme S, Faber B, Holm J, Wiklund O, Witztum JL, Hansson GK (1995) T lymphocytes from human atherosclerotic plaques recognize oxidized low density lipoprotein. *Proc Natl Acad Sci USA* 92: 3893–3897
62 Kishikawa H, Shimokama T, Watanabe T (1993) Localization of T lymphocytes and macrophages expressing IL-1, IL-2 receptor, IL-6 and TNF in human aortic intima. Role of cell-mediated immunity in human atherogenesis. *Virchows Arch A Pathol Anat Histopathol* 423: 433–442
63 Frostegard J, Ulfgren AK, Nyberg P, Hedin U, Swedenborg J, Andersson U, Hansson GK (1999) Cytokine expression in advanced human atherosclerotic plaques: dominance of pro-inflammatory (Th1) and macrophage-stimulating cytokines. *Atherosclerosis* 145: 33–43
64 Emeson EE, Shen ML, Bell CG, Qureshi A (1996) Inhibition of atherosclerosis in CD4 T-cell-ablated and nude (nu/nu) C57BL/6 hyperlipidemic mice. *Am J Pathol* 149: 675–685
65 Dansky HM, Charlton SA, Harper MM, Smith JD (1997) T and B lymphocytes play a minor role in atherosclerotic plaque formation in the apolipoprotein E-deficient mouse. *Proc Natl Acad Sci USA* 94: 4642–4646
66 Schmitz G, Herr AS, Rothe G (1998) T-lymphocytes and monocytes in atherogenesis. *Herz* 23: 168–177

67 Seko Y, Sato O, Takagi A, Tada Y, Matsuo H, Yagita H, Okumura K, Yazaki Y (1997) Perforin-secreting killer cell infiltration in the aortic tissue of patients with atherosclerotic aortic aneurysm. *Jpn Circ J* 61: 965–970
68 Zhou X, Hansson GK (1999) Detection of B cells and proinflammatory cytokines in atherosclerotic plaques of hypercholesterolemic apolipoprotein E knockout mice. *Scand J Immunol* 50: 25–30
69 Kwak B, Mulhaupt F, Myit S, Mach F (2000) Statins as a newly recognized type of immunomodulator. *Nat Med* 6: 1399–1402
70 Arita S, Une S, Ohtsuka S, Atiya A, Kasraie A, Shevlin L, Mullen Y (1998) Prevention of primary islet isograft nonfunction in mice with pravastatin. *Transplantation* 65: 1429–1433
71 Gorski A, Orlowska A, Nowaczyk M, Kasprzycka M, Rancewicz Z, Paczek L (1999) Statins inhibit T-cell interactions with elastin. *Transplant Proc* 31: 828–829
72 Montero MT, Hernandez O, Suarez Y, Matilla J, Ferruelo AJ, Martinez-Botas J, Gomez-Coronado D, Lasuncion MA (2000) Hydroxymethylglutaryl-coenzyme A reductase inhibition stimulates caspase-1 activity and Th1-cytokine release in peripheral blood mononuclear cells. *Atherosclerosis* 153: 303–313
73 Cutts JL, Scallen TJ, Watson J, Bankhurst AD (1989) Role of mevalonic acid in the regulation of natural killer cell cytotoxicity. *J Cell Physiol* 139: 550–557
74 Cutts JL, Bankhurst AD (1990) Reversal of lovastatin-mediated inhibition of natural killer cell cytotoxicity by interleukin 2. *J Cell Physiol* 145: 244–252
75 Schmitz G, Rothe G, Ruf A, Barlage S, Tschope D, Clemetson KJ, Goodall AH, Michelson AD, Nurden AT, Shankey TV (1998) European Working Group on Clinical *Cell* Analysis: Consensus protocol for the flow cytometric characterisation of platelet function. *Thromb Haemost* 79: 885–896
76 Libby P (1995) Molecular bases of the acute coronary syndromes. *Circulation* 91: 2844–2850
77 Carvalho AC, Colman RW, Lees RS (1974) Platelet function in hyperlipoproteinemia. *N Engl J Med* 290: 434–438
78 Davi G, Averna M, Catalano I, Barbagallo C, Ganci A, Notarbartolo A, Ciabattoni G, Patrono C (1992) Increased thromboxane biosynthesis in type IIa hypercholesterolemia. *Circulation* 85: 1792–1798
79 Notarbartolo A, Davi G, Averna M, Barbagallo CM, Ganci A, Giammarresi C, La Placa FP, Patrono C (1995) Inhibition of thromboxane biosynthesis and platelet function by simvastatin in type IIa hypercholesterolemia. *Arterioscler Thromb Vasc Biol* 15: 247–251
80 Song JC, White CM (2001) Do HMG-CoA reductase inhibitors affect fibrinogen? *Ann Pharmacother* 35: 236–241
81 Lacoste L, Lam JY, Hung J, Letchacovski G, Solymoss CB, Waters D (1995) Hyperlipidemia and coronary disease. Correction of the increased thrombogenic potential with cholesterol reduction. *Circulation* 92: 3172–3177
82 Aviram M, Hussein O, Rosenblat M, Schlezinger S, Hayek T, Keidar S (1998) Interactions of platelets, macrophages, and lipoproteins in hypercholesterolemia: antiatherogenic effects of HMG-CoA reductase inhibitor therapy. *J Cardiovasc Pharmacol* 31: 39–45
83 Huhle G, Abletshauser C, Mayer N, Weidinger G, Harenberg J, Heene DL (1999) Reduction of platelet activity markers in type II hypercholesterolemic patients by a HMG-CoA-reductase inhibitor. *Thromb Res* 95: 229–234
84 Szczeklik A, Musial J, Undas A, Gajewski P, Gora P, Swadzba J, Jankowski M (1999) Inhibition of thrombin generation by simvastatin and lack of additive effects of aspirin in patients with marked hypercholesterolemia. *J Am Coll Cardiol* 33: 1286–1293
85 Dangas G, Badimon JJ, Smith DA, Unger AH, Levine D, Shao JH, Meraj P, Fier C, Fallon JT, Ambrose JA (1999) Pravastatin therapy in hyperlipidemia: effects on thrombus formation and the systemic hemostatic profile. *J Am Coll Cardiol* 33: 1294–1304
86 Kearney D, Fitzgerald D (1999) The anti-thrombotic effects of statins. *J Am Coll Cardiol* 33: 1305–1307
87 Fenton JW (1981) Thrombin specificity. *Ann N Y Acad Sci* 370: 468–495
88 Fenton JW, Ofosu FA, Brezniak DV, Hassouna HI (1993) Understanding thrombin and hemostasis. *Hematol Oncol Clin North Am* 7: 1107–1119
89 Fenton JW (1995) Thrombin functions and antithrombotic intervention. *Thromb Haemost* 74: 493–498
90 Fenton JW, Ofosu FA, Brezniak DV, Hassouna HI (1998) Thrombin and antithrombotics. *Semin Thromb Hemost* 24: 87–91

91 Connolly AJ, Ishihara H, Kahn ML, Farese RVJ, Coughlin SR (1996) Role of the thrombin receptor in development and evidence for a second receptor. *Nature* 381: 516–519

92 Maltese WA (1990) Posttranslational modification of proteins by isoprenoids in mammalian cells. *FASEB J* 4: 3319–3328

93 Cichowski K, McCormick F, Brugge JS (1992) p21rasGAP association with Fyn, Lyn, and Yes in thrombin-activated platelets. *J Biol Chem* 267: 5025–5028

94 Ferro D, Basili S, Alessandri C, Mantovani B, Cordova C, Violi F (1997) Simvastatin reduces monocyte-tissue-factor expression type IIa hypercholesterolaemia. *Lancet* 350: 1222

95 Brand K, Banka CL, Mackman N, Terkeltaub RA, Fan ST, Curtiss LK (1994) Oxidized LDL enhances lipopolysaccharide-induced tissue factor expression in human adherent monocytes. *Arterioscler Thromb* 14: 790–797

96 Colli S, Eligini S, Lalli M, Camera M, Paoletti R, Tremoli E (1997) Vastatins inhibit tissue factor in cultured human macrophages. A novel mechanism of protection against atherothrombosis. *Arterioscler Thromb Vasc Biol* 17: 265–272

97 Aikawa M, Rabkin E, Sugiyama S, Voglic SJ, Fukumoto Y, Furukawa Y, Shiomi M, Schoen FJ, Libby P (2001) An HMG-CoA reductase inhibitor, cerivastatin, suppresses growth of macrophages expressing matrix metalloproteinases and tissue factor *in vivo* and *in vitro*. *Circulation* 103: 276–283

98 Aikawa M, Voglic SJ, Sugiyama S, Rabkin E, Taubman MB, Fallon JT, Libby P (1999) Dietary lipid lowering reduces tissue factor expression in rabbit atheroma. *Circulation* 100: 1215–1222

99 Crutchley DJ, Que BG (1995) Copper-induced tissue factor expression in human monocytic THP-1 cells and its inhibition by antioxidants. *Circulation* 92: 238–243

100 Le Quan S, Levenson J, Megnien JL, Simon A, Devynck MA (1995) Platelet cytosolic Ca^{2+} and membrane dynamics in patients with primary hypercholesterolemia. Effects of pravastatin. *Arterioscler Thromb Vasc Biol* 15: 759–764

101 Thomas M, Mann J (1998) Increased thrombotic vascular events after change of statin. *Lancet* 352: 1830–1831

102 Gonzalez-Ponte ML, Gonzalez-Ruiz M, Duvos E, Gutierrez-Iniguez MA, Olalla JI, Conde E (1998) Atorvastatin-induced severe thrombocytopenia. *Lancet* 352: 1284

103 McCarthy LJ, Porcu P, Fausel CA, Sweeney CJ, Danielson CF (1998) Thrombotic thrombocytopenic purpura and simvastatin. *Lancet* 352: 1284–1285

104 Zambrana JL, Velasco F, Castro P, Concha M, Valles F, Montilla P, Jimenez-Pereperez JA, Lopez-Miranda J, Perez-Jimenez F (1997) Comparison of bezafibrate *versus* lovastatin for lowering plasma insulin, fibrinogen, and plasminogen activator inhibitor-1 concentrations in hyperlipemic heart transplant patients. *Am J Cardiol* 80: 836–840

105 Wada H, Mori Y, Kaneko T, Wakita Y, Nakase T, Minamikawa K, Ohiwa M, Tamaki S, Tanigawa M, Kageyama S (1993) Elevated plasma levels of vascular endothelial cell markers in patients with hypercholesterolemia. *Am J Hematol* 44: 112–116

106 Bourcier T, Libby P (2000) HMG CoA reductase inhibitors reduce plasminogen activator inhibitor-1 expression by human vascular smooth muscle and endothelial cells. *Arterioscler Thromb Vasc Biol* 20: 556–562

107 Isaacsohn JL, Setaro JF, Nicholas C, Davey JA, Diotalevi LJ, Christianson DS, Liskov E, Stein EA, Black HR (1994) Effects of lovastatin therapy on plasminogen activator inhibitor-1 antigen levels. *Am J Cardiol* 74: 735–737

108 Davidson M, McKenney J, Stein E, Schrott H, Bakker-Arkema R, Fayyad R, Black D (1997) Comparison of one-year efficacy and safety of atorvastatin *versus* lovastatin in primary hypercholesterolemia. Atorvastatin Study Group I. *Am J Cardiol* 79: 1475–1481

109 Wada H, Mori Y, Kaneko T, Wakita Y, Minamikawa K, Ohiwa M, Tamaki S, Yokoyama N, Kobayashi T, Deguchi K (1992) Hypercoagulable state in patients with hypercholesterolemia: effects of pravastatin. *Clin Ther* 14: 829–834

110 Mitropoulos KA, Armitage JM, Collins R, Meade TW, Reeves BE, Wallendszus KR, Wilson SS, Lawson A, Peto R (1997) Randomized placebo-controlled study of the effects of simvastatin on haemostatic variables, lipoproteins and free fatty acids. The Oxford Cholesterol Study Group. *Eur Heart J* 18: 235–241

111 Bevilacqua M, Bettica P, Milani M, Vago T, Rogolino A, Righini V, Santoli E, Norbiato G (1997) Effect of fluvastatin on lipids and fibrinolysis in coronary artery disease. *Am J Cardiol* 79: 84–87

112 Koh KK, Cardillo C, Bui MN, Hathaway L, Csako G, Waclawiw MA, Panza JA, Cannon RO

(1999) Vascular effects of estrogen and cholesterol-lowering therapies in hypercholesterolemic postmenopausal women. *Circulation* 99: 354–360
113 Weiner LM, Li W, Holmes M, Catalano RB, Dovnarsky M, Padavic K, Alpaugh RK (1994) Phase I trial of recombinant macrophage colony-stimulating factor and recombinant gamma-interferon: toxicity, monocytosis, and clinical effects. *Cancer Res* 54: 4084–4090
114 Schmid I, Baldwin GC, Jacobs EL, Isacescu V, Neagos N, Giorgi JV, Glaspy JA (1995) Alterations in phenotype and cell-surface antigen expression levels of human monocytes: differential response to *in vivo* administration of rhM-CSF or rhGM-CSF. *Cytometry* 22: 103–110
115 Vanham G, Edmonds K, Qing L, Hom D, Toossi Z, Jones B, Daley CL, Huebner B, Kestens L, Gigase P et al (1996) Generalized immune activation in pulmonary tuberculosis: co-activation with HIV infection. *Clin Exp Immunol* 103: 30–34
116 Saleh MN, Goldman SJ, LoBuglio AF, Beall AC, Sabio H, McCord MC, Minasian L, Alpaugh RK, Weiner LM, Munn DH (1995) $CD16^+$ monocytes in patients with cancer: spontaneous elevation and pharmacologic induction by recombinant human macrophage colony-stimulating factor. *Blood* 85: 2910–2917
117 Nockher WA, Bergmann L, Scherberich JE (1994) Increased soluble CD14 serum levels and altered CD14 expression of peripheral blood monocytes in HIV-infected patients. *Clin Exp Immunol* 98: 369–374
118 Allen JB, Wong HL, Guyre PM, Simon GL, Wahl SM (1991) Association of circulating receptor Fc gamma RIII-positive monocytes in AIDS patients with elevated levels of transforming growth factor-beta. *J Clin Invest* 87: 1773–1779
119 Steinberg D, Parthasarathy S, Carew TE, Khoo JC, Witztum JL (1989) Beyond cholesterol. Modifications of low-density lipoprotein that increase its atherogenicity. *N Engl J Med* 320: 915–924
120 Steinberg D (1997) Lewis A. Conner Memorial Lecture. Oxidative modification of LDL and atherogenesis. *Circulation* 95: 1062–1071
121 Colles SM, Irwin KC, Chisolm GM (1996) Roles of multiple oxidized LDL lipids in cellular injury: dominance of 7 beta-hydroperoxycholesterol. *J Lipid Res* 37: 2018–2028
122 Goldstein JL, Ho YK, Basu SK, Brown MS (1979) Binding site on macrophages that mediates uptake and degradation of acetylated low density lipoprotein, producing massive cholesterol deposition. *Proc Natl Acad Sci USA* 76: 333–337
123 Bhakdi S, Dorweiler B, Kirchmann R, Torzewski J, Weise E, Tranum-Jensen J, Walev I, Wieland E (1998) On the pathogenesis of atherosclerosis: enzymatic transformation of human low density lipoprotein to an atherogenic moiety. *J Exp Med* 182: 1959–1971
124 Boren J, Olin K, Lee I, Chait A, Wight TN, Innerarity TL (1998) Identification of the principal proteoglycan-binding site in LDL. A single-point mutation in apo-B100 severely affects proteoglycan interaction without affecting LDL receptor binding. *J Clin Invest* 101: 2658–2664
125 Aviram M, Maor I, Keidar S, Hayek T, Oiknine J, Bar-El Y, Adler Z, Kertzman V, Milo S (1995) Lesioned low density lipoprotein in atherosclerotic apolipoprotein E-deficient transgenic mice and in humans is oxidized and aggregated. *Biochem Biophys Res Commun* 216: 501–513
126 Frank JS, Fogelman AM (1989) Ultrastructure of the intima in WHHL and cholesterol-fed rabbit aortas prepared by ultra-rapid freezing and freeze-etching. *J Lipid Res* 30: 967–978
127 Schissel SL, Jiang X, Tweedie-Hardman J, Jeong T, Camejo EH, Najib J, Rapp JH, Williams KJ, Tabas I (1998) Secretory sphingomyelinase, a product of the acid sphingomyelinase gene, can hydrolyze atherogenic lipoproteins at neutral pH. Implications for atherosclerotic lesion development. *J Biol Chem* 273: 2738–2746
128 Suits AG, Chait A, Aviram M, Heinecke JW (1989) Phagocytosis of aggregated lipoprotein by macrophages: low density lipoprotein receptor-dependent foam-cell formation. *Proc Natl Acad Sci USA* 86: 2713–2717
129 Bucala R, Makita Z, Koschinsky T, Cerami A, Vlassara H (1993) Lipid advanced glycosylation: pathway for lipid oxidation *in vivo*. *Proc Natl Acad Sci USA* 90: 6434–6438
130 Wang X, Bucala R, Milne R (1998) Epitopes close to the apolipoprotein B low density lipoprotein receptor-binding site are modified by advanced glycation end products. *Proc Natl Acad Sci USA* 95: 7643–7647
131 Wen FQ, Jabbar AA, Patel DA, Kazarian T, Valentino LA (1999) Atherosclerotic aortic gangliosides enhance integrin-mediated platelet adhesion to collagen. *Arterioscler Thromb Vasc Biol* 19: 519–524
132 Brandes RP, Behra A, Lebherz C, Boger RH, Bode-Boger SM, Mugge A (1999) Lovastatin main-

tains nitric oxide – but not EDHF-mediated endothelium-dependent relaxation in the hypercholesterolemic rabbit carotid artery. *Atherosclerosis* 142: 97–104
133 Endres M, Laufs U, Huang Z, Nakamura T, Huang P, Moskowitz MA, Liao JK (1998) Stroke protection by 3-hydroxy-3-methylglutaryl (HMG)-CoA reductase inhibitors mediated by endothelial nitric oxide synthase. *Proc Natl Acad Sci USA* 95: 8880–8885
134 Essig M, Nguyen G, Prie D, Escoubet B, Sraer JD, Friedlander G (1998) 3-Hydroxy-3-methylglutaryl coenzyme A reductase inhibitors increase fibrinolytic activity in rat aortic endothelial cells. Role of geranylgeranylation and Rho proteins. *Circ Res* 83: 683–690
135 Hernandez-Perera O, Perez-Sala D, Navarro-Antolin J, Sanchez-Pascuala R, Hernandez G, Diaz C, Lamas S (1998) Effects of the 3-hydroxy-3-methylglutaryl-CoA reductase inhibitors, atorvastatin and simvastatin, on the expression of endothelin-1 and endothelial nitric oxide synthase in vascular endothelial cells. *J Clin Invest* 101: 2711–2719
136 Laufs U, La Fata V, Plutzky J, Liao JK (1998) Upregulation of endothelial nitric oxide synthase by HMG CoA reductase inhibitors. *Circulation* 97: 1129–1135
137 Farnier M, Davignon J (1998) Current and future treatment of hyperlipidemia: the role of statins. *Am J Cardiol* 82: 3J–10J
138 Kreuzer J, Bader J, Jahn L, Hautmann M, Kubler W, Von Hodenberg E (1991) Chemotaxis of the monocyte cell line U937: dependence on cholesterol and early mevalonate pathway products. *Atherosclerosis* 90: 203–209
139 Muldoon MF, Flory JD, Marsland A, Manuck SB, Whiteside TL, Rabin B (1997) Effects of lovastatin on the immune system. *Am J Cardiol* 80: 1391–1394
140 Corsini A, Arnaboldi L, Raiteri M, Quarato P, Faggiotto A, Paoletti R, Fumagalli R (1996) Effect of the new HMG-CoA reductase inhibitor cerivastatin (BAY W 6228) on migration, proliferation and cholesterol synthesis in arterial myocytes. *Pharmacol Res* 33: 55–61
141 Muller C, Kiehl MG, van de Loo J, Koch OM (1999) Lovastatin induces p21WAF1/Cip1 in human vascular smooth muscle cells: influence on protein phosphorylation, cell cycle, induction of apoptosis, and growth inhibition. *Int J Mol Med* 3: 63–68
142 Vrtovsnik F, Couette S, Prie D, Lallemand D, Friedlander G (1997) Lovastatin-induced inhibition of renal epithelial tubular cell proliferation involves a p21ras activated, AP-1-dependent pathway. *Kidney Int* 52: 1016–1027
143 Fisher JE, Rogers MJ, Halasy JM, Luckman SP, Hughes DE, Masarachia PJ, Wesolowski G, Russell RG, Rodan GA, Reszka AA (1999) Alendronate mechanism of action: geranylgeraniol, an intermediate in the mevalonate pathway, prevents inhibition of osteoclast formation, bone resorption, and kinase activation *in vitro*. *Proc Natl Acad Sci USA* 96: 133–138
144 Dimitroulakos J, Nohynek D, Backway KL, Hedley DW, Yeger H, Freedman MH, Minden MD, Penn LZ (1999) Increased sensitivity of acute myeloid leukemias to lovastatin-induced apoptosis: A potential therapeutic approach. *Blood* 93: 1308–1318
145 Hunakova L, Sedlak J, Sulikova M, Chovancova J, Duraj J, Chorvath B (1997) Human multidrug-resistant (MRP,p190) myeloid leukemia HL-60/ADR cells *in vitro*: resistance to the mevalonate pathway inhibitor lovastatin. *Neoplasma* 44: 366–369
146 Lee SJ, Ha MJ, Lee J, Nguyen P, Choi YH, Pirnia F, Kang WK, Wang XF, Kim SJ, Trepel JB (1998) Inhibition of the 3-hydroxy-3-methylglutaryl-coenzyme A reductase pathway induces p53-independent transcriptional regulation of p21(WAF1/CIP1) in human prostate carcinoma cells. *J Biol Chem* 273: 10618–10623
147 Marcelli M, Cunningham GR, Haidacher SJ, Padayatty SJ, Sturgis L, Kagan C, Denner L (1998) Caspase-7 is activated during lovastatin-induced apoptosis of the prostate cancer cell line LNCaP. *Cancer Res* 58: 76–83
148 Rao S, Lowe M, Herliczek TW, Keyomarsi K (1998) Lovastatin mediated G1 arrest in normal and tumor breast cells is through inhibition of CDK2 activity and redistribution of p21 and p27, independent of p53. *Oncogene* 17: 2393–2402
149 Rubins JB, Greatens T, Kratzke RA, Tan AT, Polunovsky VA, Bitterman P (1998) Lovastatin induces apoptosis in malignant mesothelioma cells. *Am J Respir Crit Care Med* 157: 1616–1622

HMG-CoA Reductase Inhibitors
ed. by G. Schmitz and M. Torzewski

Pleiotropic effects of HMG-CoA reductase inhibitors on cells of the vascular wall

Koichi Node[1] and James K. Liao[2]

[1] *Department of Internal Medicine and Therapeutics, Osaka University Graduate School of Medicine, 2-2, Yamadaoka, Suita, Osaka 565-0871, Japan*
[2] *Department of Medicine, Brigham & Women's Hospital and Harvard Medical School, 65 Landsdowne Street, Cambridge, Massachusetts 02139, USA*

Discovery of statins

Cholesterol is an essential component of cell membranes and is the immediate precursor of steroid hormones and bile acids. However, in excessive amounts, cholesterol becomes an important risk factor for cardiovascular disease, as demonstrated in clinical trials from the Framingham Heart Study [1–3] and the Multiple Risk Factor Intervention Trial [4, 5]. Although dietary cholesterol can contribute to changes in serum cholesterol levels, more than two-thirds of the body's cholesterol is synthesized in the liver. Therefore, inhibition of hepatic cholesterol biosynthesis has emerged as the therapeutic target of choice for reducing serum cholesterol levels. The rate-limiting enzyme in cholesterol biosynthesis in the liver is 3-hydroxy-3-methylglutaryl-coenzyme A (HMG-CoA) reductase [6], which catalyzes the conversion of HMG-CoA to mevalonic acid [7] (Fig. 1).

Inhibitors of HMG-CoA reductase or statins were originally identified as secondary metabolites of fungi [8]. One of the first natural inhibitors of HMG-CoA reductase was mevastatin (compactin, ML-236B), which was isolated from *Penicillium citrinium* by A. Endo et al. in 1976 [9]. In its active form, mevastatin resembles the cholesterol precursor, HMG-CoA. When mevastatin was initially administered to rats, it inhibited cholesterol biosynthesis with a K_i of 1.4 nM. Unfortunately, it also caused unacceptable hepatocellular toxicity and further development for human use was discontinued. Subsequently, a more active fungal metabolite, mevinolin or lovastatin, was isolated from *Aspergillus terreus* by Hoffman and colleagues in 1979 [10, 11]. Lovastatin differs from mevastatin in having a substituted methyl group. Compared to mevastatin, lovastatin was a more potent inhibitor of HMG-CoA reductase with a K_i of 0.6 nM, but did not cause hepatocellular toxicity when given to rats. Lovastatin, therefore, became the first of this class of cholesterol-lowering agents to be approved for clinical use in humans. Since then, several new

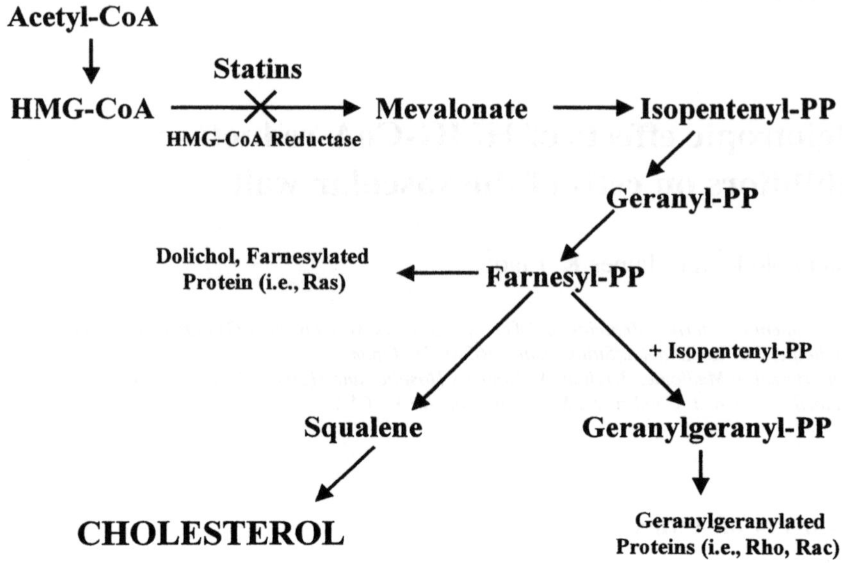

Figure 1. Cholesterol biosynthetic pathway. Inhibition of HMG-CoA reductase by statins decreases the synthesis of isoprenoids and cholesterol.

statins, both natural and chemically modified, have become commercially available, including pravastatin, simvastatin, fluvastatin, atorvastatin, cerivasatin and, most recently, pitavastatin and rosuvastatin [12]. Indeed, statins have emerged as one of the most effective classes of agents for reducing serum cholesterol levels.

Pharmacological properties of statins

Statins work by reversibly inhibiting HMG-CoA reductase through side chains that bind to the enzyme's active site and block the substrate-product transition state of the enzyme [13]. Statins bind to mammalian HMG-CoA reductase at nanomolar concentrations, leading to effective displacement of the natural substrate, HMG-CoA, which binds at micromolar concentrations [14]. Oral administration of statins to rodents and dogs showed that these drugs are predominantly extracted by the liver and resulted in >30–50% reduction in plasma total cholesterol levels and substantial decrease in urinary and plasma levels of mevalonic acid, the endproduct of the HMG-CoA reductase reaction. Similar reduction in cholesterol synthesis and decrease in circulating total and low-density lipoprotein (LDL)-containing cholesterol by these agents have been subsequently confirmed in humans. Because hepatic LDL receptors are the major mechanism of LDL clearance from the circulation, the substantial declines in serum cholesterol levels are accompanied by an increase in hepatic LDL receptor activity. Statins, therefore, effectively reduce serum cholesterol levels by two separate mechanisms. They not only inhibit endogenous cholesterol biosynthesis via HMG-CoA reductase inhibition, but they also increase cholesterol clearance from the bloodstream via increases in the LDL receptor.

The rank potency for HMG-CoA reductase inhibition among the second-generation statins are: simvastatin > pravastatin > lovastatin ≅ mevastatin with tissue IC_{50} values of simvastatin and mevastatin being approximately 4 nM and 20 nM, respectively [15]. The IC_{50} values for these statins correspond to their relative potency for lowering serum cholesterol levels *in vivo* (i.e., simvastatin > lovastatin) [16]. The newer third-generation synthetic statins, which include fluvastatin, cerivastatin, the penta-substituted pyrrole atorvastatin, pitavastatin (NK-104), and rosuvastatin, are found to be much more potent than the mevastatin derivatives. These newer statins are active compounds, which share some physico-chemical properties with pravastatin, but have greater lipophilicity and half-life [17]. Consequently, these statins, especially atorvastatin, pitavastatin, and rosuvastatin, appear to be extremely effective in lowering serum cholesterol levels, perhaps due, in part, to their ability to bind hepatic HMG-CoA reductase at higher affinity and inhibit the enzyme for a longer duration.

Because statins differ in their tissue permeability and metabolism, they possess different potencies for extra-hepatic HMG-CoA reductase inhibition. These differences in tissue permeability and metabolisms may account for some of the observed differences in their peripheral side-effects [18]. For example, the lipophilic statins are highly membrane-permeable by passive diffusion and would be expected to exert more peripheral effects than the non-permeable hydrophilic statin. These differences in cellular permeability may explain the greater incidence of peripheral myopathies observed with lipophilic statins compared to that of hydrophilic statins. Ironically, the ability of lipophilic statins to penetrate extra-hepatic cells may also make these statins more potent in terms of exerting pleiotropic effects on the vascular wall.

Clinical trials with statins

Atherosclerosis is the underlying disorder in the majority of patients with cardiovascular disease [19]. Although the development of atherosclerosis is dependent upon many factors and processes, a clear association has been established between elevated serum cholesterol levels and increased atherosclerotic disease [1–3, 5]. Recent large clinical trials have demonstrated that statins decrease the incidence of coronary heart disease in patients with hypercholesterolemia and atherosclerosis [20–24]. Depending on the dose and the type of the statin used, LDL was decreased anywhere from 19 to 60 percent in response to therapy. In addition, high-density lipoprotein (HDL) cholesterol levels were increased, and triglycerides were decreased as a result of statin therapy. These lipid effects of statins are believed to slow the progression of atherosclerosis, since atherosclerosis is mediated, in part, by the uptake of modified LDL into arteries [25]. Indeed, the importance of lowering plasma LDL levels for the prevention of coronary events is both well known and widely accepted among clinicians, with statin therapy as the current treatment of choice [26].

Because serum cholesterol level is strongly associated with coronary atherosclerotic disease [27], it has been generally assumed that cholesterol reduction by statins is the predominant, if not the only, mechanism underlying their beneficial effects in cardiovascular diseases. However, subgroup analyses of large clinical trials have challenged this notion and suggested that the beneficial effects of statins may extend to mechanisms beyond cholesterol reduction. For example, subgroup analysis of the West of Scotland Coronary Prevention (WOSCOP) and Cholesterol And Recurrent Events (CARE) studies indicates that despite comparable serum cholesterol levels among the statin-treated and placebo groups, statin-treated individuals have significantly lower risks for coronary heart disease compared to age-matched placebo-controlled individuals [22, 23, 28, 29]. Furthermore, meta-analyses of cholesterol-lowering trials suggest that the risk of myocardial infarctions in individuals treated with statins is significantly lower compared to individuals treated with other cholesterol-lowering agents or modalities despite comparable reduction in serum cholesterol levels in both groups [30, 31]. These findings suggest that statins may have beneficial effects beyond cholesterol lowering.

Further evidence in support of the non-cholesterol benefits of statin therapy is provided by angiographic trials, which demonstrated clinical improvements with statins that far exceed changes in the size of atherosclerotic lesions. For example, in the FATS trial, statin therapy with bile acid resin decreased the incidence of coronary events by 70% despite producing only a 0.7% change in lesion regression [30, 32]. Indeed, much of the beneficial effects of statins in this trial were attributed to plaque stabilization and remodeling. However, in the recent Myocardial Ischemia Reduction with Aggressive Cholesterol Lowering (MIRACL) trial, statins were found to be effective in reducing recurrent ischemic events as early as 16 weeks following acute coronary ischemia [33]. Although the serum LDL-cholesterol was reduced by 40%, this time frame was probably too short for appreciable changes in lesion size and plaque stability. Therefore, it is widely believed that some other actions of statins, particularly the improvement of endothelial function, may have contributed to these early benefits [34, 35]. Taken together, these findings suggest that the clinical benefits of statin therapy may extend beyond cholesterol lowering to include direct cellular effects on the vascular wall.

Statins and isoprenylated proteins

By inhibiting L-mevalonic acid synthesis, statins also prevent the synthesis of other important isoprenoid intermediates of the cholesterol biosynthetic pathway, such as farnesylpyrophosphate (FPP) and geranylgeranylpyrophosphate (GGPP) [6]. These intermediates serve as important lipid attachments for the post-translational modification of a variety of proteins, including the γ subunit of heterotrimeric G-proteins, Heme-a, nuclear lamins, and the small GTP-binding protein Ras, and Ras-like proteins, such as Rho, Rab, Rac, Ral or Rap [36]. Thus, protein isoprenylation permits the covalent attachment, subcellular localization, and intracellular trafficking of membrane-associated proteins. Members of the Ras and Rho GTPase family are major substrates for post-translational modification by prenylation [36, 37]. Both Ras and Rho are small GTP-binding proteins, which cycle between the inactive GDP-bound state and active GTP-bound state. In endothelial cells, Ras translocation from the cytoplasm to the plasma membrane is dependent upon farnesylation while Rho translocation is dependent upon geranylgeranylation [38, 39]. Statins inhibit both Ras and Rho isoprenylation, leading to the accumulation of inactive Ras and Rho in the cytoplasm.

Because Rho is a major target of geranylgeranylation, inhibition of Rho and its downstream target, Rho kinase, is a likely mechanism mediating some of the pleiotropic effects of statins on the vascular wall [40]. Each member of the Rho family serves specific functions in terms of cell shape, motility, secretion, and proliferation, although overlapping functions between the members could be observed in overexpressed systems. The activation of Rho in Swiss 3 T3 fibroblasts by extracellular ligands, such as platelet-derived lysophosphatidic acid, leads to myosin light chain phosphorylation and formation of focal adhesion complexes [36, 37, 41]. Indeed, Rho-associated protein kinase increases the sensitivity of vascular smooth muscle to calcium in hypertension [42] and coronary spasm [43]. In contrast, activation of Rac leads to the formation of lamellipodia and membrane ruffles, while activation of Cdc42 induces actin-rich surface protrusions called filopodia. These distinct but complementary functions of Rho family members also extend to their effects on cell signaling. When cells undergo reorganization of their actin cytoskeleton in response to extracellular signals such as growth factors or during cell movement and mitosis, they alter the three-dimensional co-localization of intracellular proteins [36, 37]. Thus, changes in the Rho-induced actin cytoskeleton can affect intracellular transport, membrane trafficking, mRNA stability, and gene transcription. It is therefore not too surprising to find that Rho-induced changes in the actin cytoskeleton and gene expression are related. Indeed, evidence suggests that inhibition of Rho isoprenylation mediates many of the cholesterol-independent effects of statins not only in vascular wall cells [38, 44], but also in leukocytes [45] and bone [46].

Statins and endothelial function

The vascular endothelium serves as an important autocrine and paracrine organ that regulates vascular wall contractile state and cellular composition.

Hypercholesterolemia impairs endothelial function and endothelial dysfunction is one of the earliest manifestations of atherosclerosis, occurring even in the absence of angiographic evidence of disease [47, 48]. An important characteristic of endothelial dysfunction is the impaired synthesis, release and activity of endothelial-derived nitric oxide (NO). Endothelial NO has been shown to inhibit several components of the atherogenic process. For example, endothelium-derived NO mediates vascular relaxation [49] and inhibits platelet aggregation [50], vascular smooth muscle proliferation [51] and endothelial-leukocyte interactions [52, 53]. Inactivation of NO by the superoxide anion ($O_2\cdot^-$) limits the bioavailability of NO and leads to nitrate tolerance, vasoconstriction, and hypertension [54, 55].

Acute plasma LDL apheresis improves endothelium-dependent vasodilation [56], suggesting that statins could restore endothelial function, in part, by lowering serum cholesterol levels. However, in some studies with statins, restoration of endothelial function occurs before significant reduction in serum cholesterol levels [57–59], suggesting that there are additional effects on endothelial function beyond that of cholesterol reduction. Indeed, statins increase endothelial NO production by stimulating and upregulating endothelial nitric oxide synthase (eNOS) [38, 60]. Furthermore, statins have been shown to restore eNOS activity in the presence of hypoxia [61] and oxidized low-density lipoprotein (ox-LDL) [38], conditions which lead to endothelial dysfunction. Statins also increase the expression of tissue-type plasminogen activator (t-PA) [62] and inhibit the expression of endothelin-1, a potent vasoconstrictor and mitogen [63]. Statins, therefore, exert many favorable effects on the endothelium and attenuate endothelial dysfunction in the presence of atherosclerotic risk factors.

While the effects of statins on Ras and Rho isoprenylation are reversed in the presence of FPP and GGPP, respectively, the effects of statins on eNOS expression is only reversed with GGPP and not by FPP or LDL-cholesterol [39]. Indeed, direct inhibition of geranylgeranyltransferase or Rho leads to increases in eNOS expression [39, 40, 64] (Fig. 2). These findings are consistent with a non-cholesterol-lowering effect of statins and suggest that inhibition of Rho by statins mediates the increase in eNOS expression. Indeed, statins upregulate eNOS expression by prolonging eNOS mRNA half-life but not eNOS gene transcription [39]. Since hypoxia, oxidized LDL, and cytokines such as TNF-α decrease eNOS expression by reducing eNOS mRNA stability, the ability of statins to prolong eNOS half-life may make them effective agents in counteracting conditions which downregulate eNOS expression.

Another potential mechanism by which statins may improve endothelial function is through their antioxidant effects. For example, statins enhance endothelium-dependent relaxation by inhibiting the production of reactive oxygen species (ROS), such as superoxide and hydroxy radicals, from aortas of cholesterol-fed rabbits [65]. Although lipid lowering by itself can lower vascular oxidative stress [66, 67], some of these antioxidant effects of statins appear to be cholesterol-independent. For example, statins attenuate

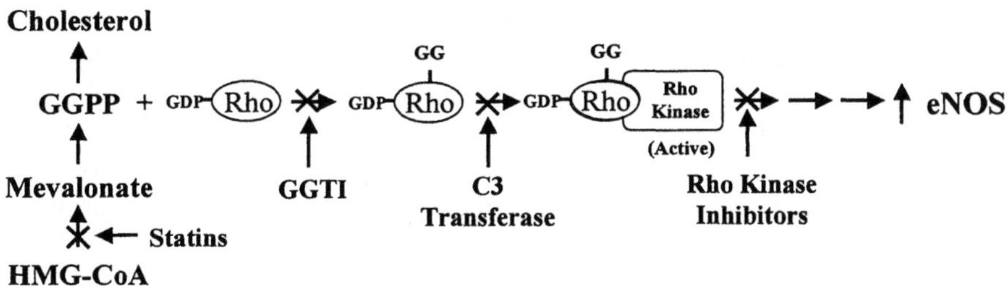

Figure 2. Regulation of eNOS expression by statins. Statins inhibit HMG-CoA reductase and block the synthesis of isoprenoids and cholesterol. The isoprenoid, geranylgeraniol (GG), is an important lipid attachment for Rho, which permits the subsequent membrane translocation and activation of Rho. Inhibition of Rho geranylgeranylation by geranylgeranyl transferase inhibitor (GGTI), Rho activity by *Clostridium botulinum* C3 transferase, or Rho kinase activity by Rho kinase inhibitors, lead to increases in eNOS expression.

angiotensin II-induced free radical production in vascular smooth muscle cells by inhibiting Rac1-mediated NADH oxidase activity and downregulating angiotensin AT1 receptor expression [68]. Since NO is scavenged by ROS, these findings indicate that the antioxidant properties of statins may also contribute to their ability to improve endothelial function [54, 55].

Statins and smooth muscle proliferation

The proliferation of vascular smooth muscle cells (SMC) is a central event in the pathogenesis of vascular lesions, including post-angioplasty restenosis, transplant arteriosclerosis and veinous graft occlusion [69]. Cellular proliferation is governed by the eukaryotic cell cycle [70], which comprises four distinct sequential phases (G_0, G_1, S, and G_2) [71]. This tightly controlled temporal order is imposed by the sequential activation of a number of serine/threonine protein kinases known as cyclin-dependent kinases (Cdks) [72], which hyperphosphorylates the retinoblastoma protein (Rb) [71]. The activity of cyclin-Cdk complexes, in turn, is negatively regulated by a number of Cdk inhibitors (CdkI) [73]. The known CdkIs can be grouped into two distinct families: the INK4 family, which includes $p16^{INK4a}$, $p15^{INK4b}$, $p18^{INK4c}$ and $p19^{INK4d}$ are specific inhibitors of Cdk-4 and Cdk-6, whereas $p21^{waf1}$/$p27^{kip1}$ family members block cell cycle progression by inhibiting cyclin D-, E-, and A-associated Cdk complexes [74].

Recent studies have shown that statins attenuate vascular proliferative disease such as transplant-associated arteriosclerosis [69]. In contrast to atherosclerosis, transplant-associated arteriosclerosis is more dependent upon immunological mechanisms, as opposed to lipid disorders, although hypercholesterolemia exacerbates the immunological process [75]. Inhibition of isoprenoid but not cholesterol synthesis by statins decreased PDGF-induced DNA synthesis in vascular SMC [44, 76]. Treatment with statins decreased PDGF-induced Rb hyperphosphorylation and cyclin-dependent kinases (cdk)-2, -4 and -6 activities. This correlated with increases in the level of Cdk inhibitor, $p27^{Kip1}$, without concomitant changes in $p16^{INK4}$, $p21^{Waf1}$, or p53 levels. These findings indicate that statins inhibit vascular SMC proliferation by arresting the cell cycle between the G1/S phase transition. It remains to be determined whether the upregulation of $p27^{Kip1}$ is responsible for the cell cycle arrest and whether there are differences between different statins in terms of $p27^{Kip1}$.

Since the small GTP-binding proteins, Ras and Rho, require post-translational modification for membrane localization and activity and are implicated in cell cycle regulation, they are likely targets for the direct anti-proliferative vascular effects of statins. Ras can promote cell cycle progression via activation of the MAP kinase pathway [77], whereas Rho causes cellular proliferation through destabilizing $p27^{Kip1}$ protein [78]. Interestingly, inhibition of vascular SMC proliferation by statins was reversed by GGPP, but not FPP or LDL-cholesterol [39]. Indeed, direct inhibition of Rho by *Clostridium botulinum* C3 transferase which ADP-ribosylates and inactivates Rho, or by a dominant-negative Rho mutant, increased $p27^{Kip1}$ and inhibited Rb hyperphosphorylation and SMC proliferation following PDGF stimulation [44]. Taken together, these findings indicate that Rho mediates PDGF-induced SMC proliferation and that inhibition of Rho by statins is the predominant mechanism by which statins inhibit vascular SMC proliferation.

Statins and platelet function

Platelets play a critical role in the development of acute coronary syndromes [79]. Circulating platelets are associated with mural thrombus formation at the site of plaque rupture and vascular injury [80–82]. Hypercholesterolemia is associated with increases in platelet reactivity [83, 84]. These abnormalities are linked to increases in the cholesterol/phospholipid ratio in platelets. Other potential mechanisms include increases in thromboxane A_2 (TXA_2) biosynthesis [85], platelet α_2-adrenergic receptor density [86], and platelet cytosolic calcium [87].

Statins have been shown to influence platelet function, although the precise mechanisms involved are not fully understood [88–90]. Potential mechanisms include a reduction in the production of TXA_2 and modifications in the cholesterol content of platelet membranes [91, 92]. The cholesterol content of platelet and erythrocyte membranes is reduced in patients taking statin therapy. This may lead to a decrease in the thrombogenic potential of these cells. Indeed, animal studies suggest statin therapy inhibits platelet deposition on damaged vessels and reduces platelet thrombus formation [81, 93, 94]. Furthermore, *in vitro* experiments have demonstrated that statins inhibit tissue factor expression by macrophages, thereby potentially reducing thrombotic events in the vascular wall [95].

Statins and plaque stability

Plaque rupture is a major cause of acute coronary syndromes [48, 96–99]. The atherosclerotic lesion contains highly thrombogenic materials in the lipid core that is separated from the bloodstream by a fibrous cap [100]. Fissuring, erosion, and ulceration of the fibrous cap eventually leads to plaque rupture and ensuing thrombosis [98]. Collagen is the main component of fibrous caps and is responsible for their tensile strength. Because macrophages are capable of degrading the collagen-containing fibrous cap, they play an important role in the development and subsequent stability of atherosclerotic plaques [101, 102]. Indeed, degradation of the plaque matrix appears to be most active in macrophage-rich regions [96, 98]. Secretion of proteolytic enzymes, such as metalloproteinases (MMPs), by activated macrophages may weaken the fibrous cap, particularly at the "vulnerable" shoulder region where the fibrous cap joins the arterial wall [103, 104]. Weakened fibrous caps lead to plaque instability, rupture and ensuing thrombosis, which ultimately present as acute coronary syndromes [99, 105].

Lipid lowering by statins may contribute to plaque stability by reducing plaque size or by modifying the physiochemical properties of the lipid core [106, 107]. However, as mentioned previously, changes in plaque size by lipid lowering tend to occur over extended time and are quite minimal as assessed by angiography. Rather, the clinical benefits from lipid lowering are probably due to decreases in macrophage accumulation in atherosclerotic lesions and inhibition of MMP production by activated macrophages [95]. Indeed, statins inhibit the expression of MMPs and tissue factor by cholesterol-dependent and –independent mechanisms [95, 106, 108], with the cholesterol-independent or direct macrophage effects occurring at a much earlier time point. The plaque-stabilizing properties of statins, therefore, are mediated through a combined reduction in lipids, macrophages, and MMPs [109]. These effects of statins may reduce the incidence of acute coronary syndromes by lessening the propensity for plaque to rupture.

Statins and vascular inflammation

Atherosclerosis is a complex inflammatory process that is characterized by the presence of monocytes or macrophages and T-lymphocytes in the atheroma [25, 110]. Inflammatory cytokines secreted by these macrophages and T-lymphocytes can modify endothelial function, SMC proliferation, collagen degradation, and thrombosis [99]. An early step in atherogenesis involves monocyte adhesion to the endothelium and penetration into the subendothelial space [110]. Recent studies suggest that statins possess anti-inflammatory properties by their ability to reduce the number of inflammatory cells in atherosclerotic plaques [91]. The mechanisms have yet to be fully elucidated, but may involve inhibition of adhesion molecules, such as intercellular adhesion molecule-1

(ICAM-1), which are involved in the recruitment of inflammatory cells [111]. Furthermore, statins attenuate P-selectin expression and leukocyte adhesion in normocholesterolemic animals by increasing endothelial NO production [112, 113]. This cholesterol-independent effect of statins was absent in eNOS-deficient mice, suggesting that eNOS mediated the vascular protective effects of statins [114].

A clinical marker of inflammation is high-sensitivity C-reactive protein (hs-CRP) [115]. hs-CRP is an acute phase reactant that is produced by the liver in response to pro-inflammatory cytokines such as interleukin-6 (IL-6) and reflects low-grade systemic inflammation [116]. Elevated levels of hs-CRP have been shown to be predictive of increased risk for coronary artery disease (CAD) in apparently healthy men and women [50, 117–120]. hs-CRP is elevated in patients with CAD, coronary ischemia and myocardial infarction compared with normal subjects [57, 121, 122]. It has been suggested that CRP could contribute to the development of atherosclerosis by binding to modified LDL within atherosclerotic plaques [123, 124]. Once CRP becomes bound, it activates complement, which has been shown to play a role in promoting atherosclerotic lesion progression [125]. However, further studies are needed to fully elucidate the role CRP plays in atherosclerosis.

Statin therapy lowers hs-CRP levels in hypercholesterolemic patients [115, 126, 127]. In the Cholesterol and Recurrent Events (CARE) trial, statins significantly decreased plasma hs-CRP levels over a 5-year period in patients who did not experience recurrent coronary events [128, 129]. Similarly, an analysis of baseline and 1-year follow-up date from the Air Force/Texas Coronary Atherosclerosis Prevention Study (AFCAPS/TexCAPS) demonstrated that hs-CRP levels were reduced in statin-treated patients who were free of acute major coronary events [115]. Futhermore, preliminary data from the Pravastatin Inflammation/CRP Evaluation (PRINCE) study confirm that statin therapy can significantly reduce serum hs-CRP levels in primary and secondary prevention populations [130]. Following 24 weeks of therapy with a statin, the hs-CRP level was reduced by approximately 13% in primary and secondary prevention populations, while placebo treatment of subjects in the primary prevention arm of the study had no effect. These studies, therefore, indicate that statins are effective in decreasing systemic and vascular inflammation. However, any potential clinical benefits conferred by the lowering of hs-CRP are difficult to separate from those of the lipid-lowering effects of statins without performing further clinical studies.

Statins and ischemic stroke

An intriguing result of large clinical trials with statins is the reduction in ischemic stroke [131]. Although myocardial infarction is closely associated with serum cholesterol levels, neither the Framingham Heart Study nor the Multiple Risk Factor Intervention Trial (MRFIT) demonstrated significant correlation between ischemic stroke and serum cholesterol levels [1, 4]. Thus, the findings of these large statin trials raise the interesting question of how a class of cholesterol-lowering agents can reduce ischemic stroke when ischemic stroke is not related to cholesterol levels. It appears likely that there are pleiotropic effects of statins, which are beneficial for ischemic stroke. Some of these beneficial effects may be attributed to the effects of statins on endothelial function and the vascular wall.

Cerebrovascular tone and blood flow are regulated by endothelium-derived NO [132]. Mutant mice lacking eNOS (eNOS$^{-/-}$) are relatively hypertensive and develop greater proliferative and inflammatory responses to vascular injury [133]. Indeed, eNOS$^{-/-}$ mice develop larger cerebral infarcts following cerebrovascular occlusion [134]. Thus, the beneficial effects of statins, in ischemic stroke may be due, in part, to their ability to upregulate eNOS expression and activity [38, 60]. For example, mice, which were prophylactically treated with statins for up to 2 weeks, have 25–30% higher cerebral blood flow and 50% smaller cerebral infarct sizes following cerebrovascular occlusion [40, 135]. No increase in cerebral blood flow or neuroprotection was observed in eNOS$^{-/-}$ mice treated with statins, indicating that the upregulation of eNOS accounts for most, if not all, of the neuroprotective effects of these agents. Interestingly, treatment with statins did not affect blood pressure or heart rate before, during, or after cerebrovascular ischemia and did not alter serum cholesterol levels in mice, consistent with the cholesterol-independent, neuroprotective effects of statins.

In addition to increases in cerebral blood flow, other beneficial effects of statins are likely to occur which can affect the severity of ischemic stroke. For example, statins attenuate P-selectin expression and leukocyte adhesion via increases in NO production in a model of cardiac ischemia and reperfusion [112, 136]. Others have reported that statins upregulate t-PA and downregulate plasminogen activator inhibitor (PAI)-1 expression through a similar mechanism involving inhibition of Rho geranylgeranylation [62]. Thus, the absence of neuroprotection in eNOS-deficient mice emphasizes the importance of endothelium-derived NO not only in augmenting cerebral blood flow, but also, potentially, in limiting the impact of platelet and white blood cell accumulation on tissue viability following ischemia. It is possible that statins may have contributed to the decrease in the incidence of ischemic strokes in clinical trials, in part, by reducing cerebral infarcts size to levels which are clinically unappreciated.

Summary

Statins exert many pleiotropic effects in addition to the lowering of serum cholesterol levels. These additional properties include beneficial effects on endothelial function and blood flow, decreasing LDL oxidation, enhancing the stability of atherosclerotic plaques, inhibiting vascular smooth muscle prolif-

Table 1. Pleiotropic effects of statins on vascular wall cells

Endothelial cells	↑ Endothelial nitric oxide synthase (eNOS) expression and activity ↑ Tissue-type plasminogen activator (t-PA) expression ↓ Plasminogen activator inhibitor-1 (PAI-1) expression ↓ Endothelin-1 synthesis and expression ↓ Reactive oxygen species ↑ Peroxisome proliferator activated receptor (PPAR)-α expression ↓ Proinflammatory cytokines (IL-1β, IL-6, cyclooxygenase-2) expression ↓ Major histocompatibility (MHC) class II antigen expression
Smooth muscle cells	↓ Migration and proliferation ↓ Reactive oxygen species ↓ Rac1-mediated NADH oxidase activity ↓ Angiotensin AT1 receptor expression ↑ Apoptosis
Platelets	↓ Platelet reactivity ↓ Thromboxane A_2 biosynthesis
Monocyte/macrophages	↓ Macrophage growth ↓ Matrix metalloproteinase (MMP) expression and secretion ↓ Tissue factor expression and activity ↓ Inducible nitric oxide synthase (iNOS) expression ↓ Proinflammatory cytokines (TNF-α, IL-1β, IL-6) expression ↓ Monocytochemoattractant protein (MCP)-1 secretion ↓ Interleukin (IL)-8 secretion ↓ Major histocompatibility (MHC) class II antigen expression
Vascular inflammation	↓ High-sensitivity C-reactive protein (hs-CRP) level ↓ Leukocyte-endothelial cell adhesion ↓ Adhesion molecule expression ↓ Nuclear factor-κB (NF-κB) activation

eration and platelet aggregation, and reducing vascular inflammation (Tab. 1). Recent evidence suggests that most of these effects are mediated by the inhibitory effect of statins on isoprenoid synthesis. In particular, inhibition of Rho GTPases in vascular wall cells by statins leads to increased expression of atheroprotective genes and inhibition of vascular smooth muscle cell proliferation. It remains to be determined which, if any, of these pleiotropic effects account for the clinical benefits of statin therapy beyond cholesterol lowering.

Acknowledgement
The work described in this paper was supported in part by the National Institutes of Health (HL-52233, HL-34836, and NS-10828) and the American Heart Association Bugher Foundation Award. Dr. Liao is an Established Investigator of the American Heart Association.

References

1 Sytkowski PA, Kannel WB, D'Agostino RB (1990) Changes in risk factors and the decline in mortality from cardiovascular disease. The Framingham Heart Study. *N Engl J Med* 322: 1635–1641
2 Gordon T, Kannel WB (1971) Premature mortality from coronary heart disease. The Framingham study. *JAMA* 215: 1617–1625

3 Kannel WB, Castelli WP, Gordon T, McNamara PM (1971) Serum cholesterol, lipoproteins, and the risk of coronary heart disease. The Framingham study. *Ann Intern Med* 74: 1–12
4 Multiple risk factor intervention trial (1982) Risk factor changes and mortality results. Multiple Risk Factor Intervention Trial Research Group. *JAMA* 248: 1465–1477
5 Iso H, Jacobs DR Jr, Wentworth D, Neaton JD, Cohen JD (1989) Serum cholesterol levels and six-year mortality from stroke in 350,977 men screened for the multiple risk factor intervention trial. *N Engl J Med* 320: 904–910
6 Goldstein JL, Brown MS (1990) Regulation of the mevalonate pathway. *Nature* 343: 425–430
7 Rodwell VW, Nordstrom JL, Mitschelen JJ (1976) Regulation of HMG-CoA reductase. *Adv Lipid Res* 14: 1–74
8 Alberts AW (1988) Discovery, biochemistry and biology of lovastatin. *Am J Cardiol* 62: 10J–15J
9 Endo A, Kuroda M, Tsujita Y (1976) ML-236A, ML-236B, and ML-236C, new inhibitors of cholesterogenesis produced by *Penicillium citrinium. J Antibiot (Tokyo)* 29: 1346–1348
10 Alberts AW, Chen J, Kuron G, Hunt V, Huff J, Hoffman C, Rothrock J, Lopez M, Joshua H, Harris E et al (1980) Mevinolin: a highly potent competitive inhibitor of hydroxymethylglutaryl-coenzyme A reductase and a cholesterol-lowering agent. *Proc Natl Acad Sci USA* 77: 3957–3961
11 Alberts AW (1990) Lovastatin and simvastatin – inhibitors of HMG CoA reductase and cholesterol biosynthesis. *Cardiology* 77: 14–21
12 Illingworth DR, Tobert JA (2001) HMG-CoA reductase inhibitors. *Adv Protein Chem* 56: 77–114
13 Istvan ES, Deisenhofer J (2001) Structural mechanism for statin inhibition of HMG-CoA reductase. *Science* 292: 1160–1164
14 Moghadasian MH (1999) Clinical pharmacology of 3-hydroxy-3-methylglutaryl coenzyme A reductase inhibitors. *Life Sci* 65: 1329–1337
15 Blum CB (1994) Comparison of properties of four inhibitors of 3-hydroxy-3- methylglutaryl-coenzyme A reductase. *Am J Cardiol* 73: 3D–11D
16 Dansette PM, Jaoen M, Pons C (2000) HMG-CoA reductase activity in human liver microsomes: comparative inhibition by statins. *Exp Toxicol Pathol* 52: 145–148
17 McTaggart F, Buckett L, Davidson R, Holdgate G, McCormick A, Schneck D, Smith G, Warwick M (2001) Preclinical and clinical pharmacology of Rosuvastatin, a new 3-hydroxy- 3-methylglutaryl coenzyme A reductase inhibitor. *Am J Cardiol* 87: 28B–32B
18 Germershausen JI, Hunt VM, Bostedor RG, Bailey PJ, Karkas JD, Alberts AW (1989) Tissue selectivity of the cholesterol-lowering agents lovastatin, simvastatin and pravastatin in rats *in vivo*. *Biochem Biophys Res Commun* 158: 667–675
19 Kastelein JJ (1999) The future of best practice. *Atherosclerosis* 143 Suppl 1: S17–21
20 (1994) Randomised trial of cholesterol lowering in 4444 patients with coronary heart disease: the Scandinavian Simvastatin Survival Study (4S). *Lancet* 344: 1383–1389
21 (1998) Prevention of cardiovascular events and death with pravastatin in patients with coronary heart disease and a broad range of initial cholesterol levels. The Long-Term Intervention with Pravastatin in Ischaemic Disease (LIPID) Study Group. *N Engl J Med* 339: 1349–1357
22 Sacks FM, Pfeffer MA, Moye LA, Rouleau JL, Rutherford JD, Cole TG, Brown L, Warnica JW, Arnold JM, Wun CC et al (1996) The effect of pravastatin on coronary events after myocardial infarction in patients with average cholesterol levels. Cholesterol and Recurrent Events Trial investigators. *N Engl J Med* 335: 1001–1009
23 Shepherd J, Cobbe SM, Ford I, Isles CG, Lorimer AR, MacFarlane PW, McKillop JH, Packard CJ (1995) Prevention of coronary heart disease with pravastatin in men with hypercholesterolemia. West of Scotland Coronary Prevention Study Group. *N Engl J Med* 333: 1301–1307
24 Downs JR, Clearfield M, Weis S, Whitney E, Shapiro DR, Beere PA, Langendorfer A, Stein EA, Kruyer W, Gotto AM Jr (1998) Primary prevention of acute coronary events with lovastatin in men and women with average cholesterol levels: results of AFCAPS/TexCAPS. Air Force/Texas Coronary Atherosclerosis Prevention Study. *JAMA* 279: 1615–1622
25 Ross R (1993) The pathogenesis of atherosclerosis: a perspective for the 1990s. *Nature* 362: 801–809
26 Maron DJ, Fazio S, Linton MF (2000) Current perspectives on statins. *Circulation* 101: 207–213
27 Klag MJ, Ford DE, Mead LA, He J, Whelton PK, Liang KY, Levine DM (1993) Serum cholesterol in young men and subsequent cardiovascular disease. *N Engl J Med* 328: 313–318
28 Massy ZA, Keane WF, Kasiske BL (1996) Inhibition of the mevalonate pathway: benefits beyond cholesterol reduction? *Lancet* 347: 102–103
29 Packard CJ (1998) Influence of pravastatin and plasma lipids on clinical events in the West of

Scotland Coronary Prevention Study (WOSCOPS). *Circulation* 97: 1440–1445
30 Brown BG, Zhao XQ, Sacco DE, Albers JJ (1993) Lipid lowering and plaque regression. New insights into prevention of plaque disruption and clinical events in coronary disease. *Circulation* 87: 1781–1791
31 Pekkanen J, Linn S, Heiss G, Suchindran CM, Leon A, Rifkind BM, Tyroler HA (1990) Ten-year mortality from cardiovascular disease in relation to cholesterol level among men with and without preexisting cardiovascular disease. *N Engl J Med* 322: 1700–1707
32 Brown BG, Hillger L, Zhao XQ, Poulin D, Albers JJ (1995) Types of change in coronary stenosis severity and their relative importance in overall progression and regression of coronary disease. Observations from the FATS Trial. Familial Atherosclerosis Treatment Study. *Ann N Y Acad Sci* 748: 407–417; discussion 417–408
33 Schwartz GG, Olsson AG, Ezekowitz MD, Ganz P, Oliver MF, Waters D, Zeiher A, Chaitman BR, Leslie S, Stern T (2001) Effects of atorvastatin on early recurrent ischemic events in acute coronary syndromes: the MIRACL study: a randomized controlled trial. *JAMA* 285: 1711–1718
34 Bellosta S, Ferri N, Bernini F, Paoletti R, Corsini A (2000) Non-lipid-related effects of statins. *Ann Med* 32: 164–176
35 Bellosta S, Ferri N, Arnaboldi L, Bernini F, Paoletti R, Corsini A (2000) Pleiotropic effects of statins in atherosclerosis and diabetes. *Diabetes Care* 23 Suppl 2: B72–78
36 Van Aelst L, D'Souza-Schorey C (1997) Rho GTPases and signaling networks. *Genes Dev* 11: 2295–2322
37 Hall A (1998) Rho GTPases and the actin cytoskeleton. *Science* 279: 509–514
38 Laufs U, La Fata V, Plutzky J, Liao JK (1998) Upregulation of endothelial nitric oxide synthase by HMG CoA reductase inhibitors. *Circulation* 97: 1129–1135
39 Laufs U, Liao JK (1998) Post-transcriptional regulation of endothelial nitric oxide synthase mRNA stability by Rho GTPase. *J Biol Chem* 273: 24266–24271
40 Laufs U, Endres M, Stagliano N, Amin-Hanjani S, Chui DS, Yang SX, Simoncini T, Yamada M, Rabkin E, Allen PG et al (2000) Neuroprotection mediated by changes in the endothelial actin cytoskeleton. *J Clin Invest* 106: 15–24
41 Hall A (1994) Small GTP-binding proteins and the regulation of the actin cytoskeleton. *Annu Rev Cell Biol* 10: 31–54
42 Uehata M, Ishizaki T, Satoh H, Ono T, Kawahara T, Morishita T, Tamakawa H, Yamagami K, Inui J, Maekawa M et al (1997) Calcium sensitization of smooth muscle mediated by a Rho-associated protein kinase in hypertension. *Nature* 389: 990–994
43 Katsumata N, Shimokawa H, Seto M, Kozai T, Yamawaki T, Kuwata K, Egashira K, Ikegaki I, Asano T, Sasaki Y et al (1997) Enhanced myosin light chain phosphorylations as a central mechanism for coronary artery spasm in a swine model with interleukin-1beta. *Circulation* 96: 4357–4363
44 Laufs U, Marra D, Node K, Liao JK (1999) 3-Hydroxy-3-methylglutaryl-CoA reductase inhibitors attenuate vascular smooth muscle proliferation by preventing rho GTPase-induced down- regulation of p27(Kip1). *J Biol Chem* 274: 21926–21931
45 Singh R, Wang B, Shirvaikar A, Khan S, Kamat S, Schelling JR, Konieczkowski M, Sedor JR (1999) The IL-1 receptor and Rho directly associate to drive cell activation in inflammation. *J Clin Invest* 103: 1561–1570
46 Mundy G, Garrett R, Harris S, Chan J, Chen D, Rossini G, Boyce B, Zhao M, Gutierrez G (1999) Stimulation of bone formation *in vitro* and in rodents by statins. *Science* 286: 1946–1949
47 Liao JK, Bettmann MA, Sandor T, Tucker JI, Coleman SM, Creager MA (1991) Differential impairment of vasodilator responsiveness of peripheral resistance and conduit vessels in humans with atherosclerosis. *Circ Res* 68: 1027–1034
48 Libby P, Sukhova G, Lee RT, Liao JK (1997) Molecular biology of atherosclerosis. *Int J Cardiol* 62 Suppl 2: S23–29
49 Ignarro LJ, Buga GM, Wood KS, Byrns RE, Chaudhuri G (1987) Endothelium-derived relaxing factor produced and released from artery and vein is nitric oxide. *Proc Natl Acad Sci USA* 84: 9265–9269
50 Radomski MW, Rees DD, Dutra A, Moncada S (1992) S-nitroso-glutathione inhibits platelet activation *in vitro* and *in vivo*. *Br J Pharmacol* 107: 745–749
51 Garg UC, Hassid A (1989) Nitric oxide-generating vasodilators and 8-bromo-cyclic guanosine monophosphate inhibit mitogenesis and proliferation of cultured rat vascular smooth muscle cells. *J Clin Invest* 83: 1774–1777

52 Gauthier TW, Scalia R, Murohara T, Guo JP, Lefer AM (1995) Nitric oxide protects against leukocyte-endothelium interactions in the early stages of hypercholesterolemia. *Arterioscler Thromb Vasc Biol* 15: 1652–1659
53 Kubes P, Suzuki M, Granger DN (1991) Nitric oxide: an endogenous modulator of leukocyte adhesion. *Proc Natl Acad Sci USA* 88: 4651–4655
54 Harrison DG (1997) Cellular and molecular mechanisms of endothelial cell dysfunction. *J Clin Invest* 100: 2153–2157
55 Munzel T, Sayegh H, Freeman BA, Tarpey MM, Harrison DG (1995) Evidence for enhanced vascular superoxide anion production in nitrate tolerance. A novel mechanism underlying tolerance and cross-tolerance. *J Clin Invest* 95: 187–194
56 Tamai O, Matsuoka H, Itabe H, Wada Y, Kohno K, Imaizumi T (1997) Single LDL apheresis improves endothelium-dependent vasodilation in hypercholesterolemic humans. *Circulation* 95: 76–82
57 Anderson TJ, Meredith IT, Yeung AC, Frei B, Selwyn AP, Ganz P (1995) The effect of cholesterol-lowering and antioxidant therapy on endothelium-dependent coronary vasomotion. *N Engl J Med* 332: 488–493
58 O`Driscoll G, Green D, Taylor RR (1997) Simvastatin, an HMG-coenzyme A reductase inhibitor, improves endothelial function within 1 month. *Circulation* 95: 1126–1131
59 Treasure CB, Klein JL, Weintraub WS, Talley JD, Stillabower ME, Kosinski AS, Zhang J, Boccuzzi SJ, Cedarholm JC, Alexander RW (1995) Beneficial effects of cholesterol-lowering therapy on the coronary endothelium in patients with coronary artery disease. *N Engl J Med* 332: 481–487
60 Kureishi Y, Luo Z, Shiojima I, Bialik A, Fulton D, Lefer DJ, Sessa WC, Walsh K (2000) The HMG-CoA reductase inhibitor simvastatin activates the protein kinase Akt and promotes angiogenesis in normocholesterolemic animals. *Nat Med* 6: 1004–1010
61 Laufs U, Fata VL, Liao JK (1997) Inhibition of 3-hydroxy-3-methylglutaryl (HMG)-CoA reductase blocks hypoxia-mediated down-regulation of endothelial nitric oxide synthase. *J Biol Chem* 272: 31725–31729
62 Essig M, Nguyen G, Prie D, Escoubet B, Sraer JD, Friedlander G (1998) 3-Hydroxy-3-methylglutaryl coenzyme A reductase inhibitors increase fibrinolytic activity in rat aortic endothelial cells. Role of geranylgeranylation and Rho proteins. *Circ Res* 83: 683–690
63 Hernandez-Perera O, Perez-Sala D, Navarro-Antolin J, Sanchez-Pascuala R, Hernandez G, Diaz C, Lamas S (1998) Effects of the 3-hydroxy-3-methylglutaryl-CoA reductase inhibitors, atorvastatin and simvastatin, on the expression of endothelin-1 and endothelial nitric oxide synthase in vascular endothelial cells. *J Clin Invest* 101: 2711–2719
64 Laufs U, Endres M, Custodis F, Gertz K, Nickenig G, Liao JK, Bohm M (2000) Suppression of endothelial nitric oxide production after withdrawal of statin treatment is mediated by negative feedback regulation of rho GTPase gene transcription. *Circulation* 102: 3104–3110
65 Rikitake Y, Kawashima S, Takeshita S, Yamashita T, Azumi H, Yasuhara M, Nishi H, Inoue N, Yokoyama M (2001) Anti-oxidative properties of fluvastatin, an HMG-CoA reductase inhibitor, contribute to prevention of atherosclerosis in cholesterol-fed rabbits. *Atherosclerosis* 154: 87–96
66 Landmesser U, Hornig B, Drexler H (2000) Endothelial dysfunction in hypercholesterolemia: mechanisms, pathophysiological importance, and therapeutic interventions. *Semin Thromb Hemost* 26: 529–537
67 Cai H, Harrison DG (2000) Endothelial dysfunction in cardiovascular diseases: the role of oxidant stress. *Circ Res* 87: 840–844
68 Wassmann S, Laufs U, Baumer AT, Muller K, Ahlbory K, Linz W, Itter G, Rosen R, Bohm M, Nickenig G (2001) HMG-CoA reductase inhibitors improve endothelial dysfunction in normocholesterolemic hypertension via reduced production of reactive oxygen species. *Hypertension* 37: 1450–1457
69 Braun-Dullaeus RC, Mann MJ, Dzau VJ (1998) *Cell* cycle progression: new therapeutic target for vascular proliferative disease. *Circulation* 98: 82–89
70 Sherr CJ (1996) Cancer cell cycles. *Science* 274: 1672–1677
71 Zetterberg A, Larsson O (1995) Cell cycle progression and cell growth in mammalian cells. *In*: C Hutchinson, DM Glover (eds): *Frontiers in Molecular Biology: Cell Cycle Control.* Oxford University Press, Oxford, pp 29–45
72 Pines J (1994) Protein kinases and cell cycle control. *Semin Cell Biol* 5: 399–408
73 Elledge SJ, Harper JW (1994) Cdk inhibitors: on the threshold of checkpoints and development. *Curr Opin Cell Biol* 6: 847–852

74 Xiong Y, Hannon GJ, Zhang H, Casso D, Kobayashi R, Beach D (1993) p21 is a universal inhibitor of cyclin kinases. *Nature* 366: 701–704
75 Kobashigawa JA, Katznelson S, Laks H, Johnson JA, Yeatman L, Wang XM, Chia D, Terasaki PI, Sabad A, Cogert GA et al (1995) Effect of pravastatin on outcomes after cardiac transplantation. *N Engl J Med* 333: 621–627
76 Yang Z, Kozai T, van der Loo B, Viswambharan H, Lachat M, Turina MI, Malinski T, Luscher TF (2000) HMG-CoA reductase inhibition improves endothelial cell function and inhibits smooth muscle cell proliferation in human saphenous veins. *J Am Coll Cardiol* 36: 1691–1697
77 Hughes DA (1995) Control of signal transduction and morphogenesis by Ras. *Semin Cell Biol* 6: 89–94
78 Hengst L, Reed SI (1996) Translational control of p27Kip1 accumulation during the cell cycle. *Science* 271: 1861–1864
79 Fitzgerald DJ, Roy L, Catella F, FitzGerald GA (1986) Platelet activation in unstable coronary disease. *N Engl J Med* 315: 983–989
80 Fuster V, Badimon JJ, Badimon L (1992) Clinical-pathological correlations of coronary disease progression and regression. *Circulation* 86: III1–11
81 Lacoste L, Lam JY, Hung J, Letchacovski G, Solymoss CB, Waters D (1995) Hyperlipidemia and coronary disease. Correction of the increased thrombogenic potential with cholesterol reduction. *Circulation* 92: 3172–3177
82 Willerson JT, Golino P, Eidt J, Campbell WB, Buja LM (1989) Specific platelet mediators and unstable coronary artery lesions. Experimental evidence and potential clinical implications. *Circulation* 80: 198–205
83 Opper C, Clement C, Schwarz H, Krappe J, Steinmetz A, Schneider J, Wesemann W (1995) Increased number of high sensitive platelets in hypercholesterolemia, cardiovascular diseases, and after incubation with cholesterol. *Atherosclerosis* 113: 211–217
84 Tremoli E, Colli S, Maderna P, Baldassarre D, Di Minno G (1993) Hypercholesterolemia and platelets. *Semin Thromb Hemost* 19: 115–121
85 Notarbartolo A, Davi G, Averna M, Barbagallo CM, Ganci A, Giammarresi C, La Placa FP, Patrono C (1995) Inhibition of thromboxane biosynthesis and platelet function by simvastatin in type IIa hypercholesterolemia. *Arterioscler Thromb Vasc Biol* 15: 247–251
86 Baldassarre D, Mores N, Colli S, Pazzucconi F, Sirtori CR, Tremoli E (1997) Platelet alpha 2-adrenergic receptors in hypercholesterolemia: relationship between binding studies and epinephrine-induced platelet aggregation. *Clin Pharmacol Ther* 61: 684–691
87 Le Quan Sang KH, Levenson J, Megnien JL, Simon A, Devynck MA (1995) Platelet cytosolic Ca^{2+} and membrane dynamics in patients with primary hypercholesterolemia. Effects of pravastatin. *Arterioscler Thromb Vasc Biol* 15: 759–764
88 Huhle G, Abletshauser C, Mayer N, Weidinger G, Harenberg J, Heene DL (1999) Reduction of platelet activity markers in type II hypercholesterolemic patients by a HMG-CoA-reductase inhibitor. *Thromb Res* 95: 229–234
89 Hale LP, Craver KT, Berrier AM, Sheffield MV, Case LD, Owen J (1998) Combination of fosinopril and pravastatin decreases platelet response to thrombin receptor agonist in monkeys. *Arterioscler Thromb Vasc Biol* 18: 1643–1646
90 Schror K (1990) Platelet reactivity and arachidonic acid metabolism in type II hyperlipoproteinaemia and its modification by cholesterol-lowering agents. *Eicosanoids* 3: 67–73
91 Vaughan CJ, Gotto AM Jr, Basson CT (2000) The evolving role of statins in the management of atherosclerosis. *J Am Coll Cardiol* 35: 1–10
92 Lijnen P, Echevaria-Vazquez D, Petrov V (1996) Influence of cholesterol-lowering on plasma membrane lipids and function. *Methods Find Exp Clin Pharmacol* 18: 123–136
93 Alfon J, Royo T, Garcia-Moll X, Badimon L (1999) Platelet deposition on eroded vessel walls at a stenotic shear rate is inhibited by lipid-lowering treatment with atorvastatin. *Arterioscler Thromb Vasc Biol* 19: 1812–1817
94 Alfon J, Fernandez de Arriba A, Gomez-Casajus LA, Merlos M (2001) Alternative binding assay of gp iib/iiia antagonists with a nonradioactive labeling method of platelets. *Thromb Res* 102: 247–253
95 Aikawa M, Rabkin E, Sugiyama S, Voglic SJ, Fukumoto Y, Furukawa Y, Shiomi M, Schoen FJ, Libby P (2001) An HMG-CoA reductase inhibitor, cerivastatin, suppresses growth of macrophages expressing matrix metalloproteinases and tissue factor *in vivo* and *in vitro*. *Circulation* 103: 276–283

96 Fuster V (1995) Elucidation of the role of plaque instability and rupture in acute coronary events. *Am J Cardiol* 76: 24C–33C
97 Chesebro JH, Zoldhelyi P, Fuster V (1991) Pathogenesis of thrombosis in unstable angina. *Am J Cardiol* 68: 2B–10B
98 Fuster V, Stein B, Ambrose JA, Badimon L, Badimon JJ, Chesebro JH (1990) Atherosclerotic plaque rupture and thrombosis. Evolving concepts. *Circulation* 82: II47–59
99 Libby P (1995) Molecular bases of the acute coronary syndromes. *Circulation* 91: 2844–2850
100 Fernandez-Ortiz A, Badimon JJ, Falk E, Fuster V, Meyer B, Mailhac A, Weng D, Shah PK, Badimon L (1994) Characterization of the relative thrombogenicity of atherosclerotic plaque components: implications for consequences of plaque rupture. *J Am Coll Cardiol* 23: 1562–1569
101 Moreno PR, Falk E, Palacios IF, Newell JB, Fuster V, Fallon JT (1994) Macrophage infiltration in acute coronary syndromes. Implications for plaque rupture. *Circulation* 90: 775–778
102 Shah PK, Falk E, Badimon JJ, Fernandez-Ortiz A, Mailhac A, Villareal-Levy G, Fallon JT, Regnstrom J, Fuster V (1995) Human monocyte-derived macrophages induce collagen breakdown in fibrous caps of atherosclerotic plaques. Potential role of matrix-degrading metalloproteinases and implications for plaque rupture. *Circulation* 92: 1565–1569
103 Henney AM, Wakeley PR, Davies MJ, Foster K, Hembry R, Murphy G, Humphries S (1991) Localization of stromelysin gene expression in atherosclerotic plaques by *in situ* hybridization. *Proc Natl Acad Sci USA* 88: 8154–8158
104 Richardson PD, Davies MJ, Born GV (1989) Influence of plaque configuration and stress distribution on fissuring of coronary atherosclerotic plaques. *Lancet* 2: 941–944
105 Davies MJ (1995) Acute coronary thrombosis – the role of plaque disruption and its initiation and prevention. *Eur Heart J* 16 Suppl L: 3–7
106 Fukumoto Y, Libby P, Rabkin E, Hill CC, Enomoto M, Hirouchi Y, Shiomi M, Aikawa M (2001) Statins alter smooth muscle cell accumulation and collagen content in established atheroma of watanabe heritable hyperlipidemic rabbits. *Circulation* 103: 993–999
107 Koh KK (2000) Effects of statins on vascular wall: vasomotor function, inflammation, and plaque stability. *Cardiovasc Res* 47: 648–657
108 Bourcier T, Libby P (2000) HMG CoA reductase inhibitors reduce plasminogen activator inhibitor-1 expression by human vascular smooth muscle and endothelial cells. *Arterioscler Thromb Vasc Biol* 20: 556–562
109 Crisby M, Nordin-Fredriksson G, Shah PK, Yano J, Zhu J, Nilsson J (2001) Pravastatin treatment increases collagen content and decreases lipid content, inflammation, metalloproteinases, and cell death in human carotid plaques: implications for plaque stabilization. *Circulation* 103: 926–933
110 Ross R (1999) Atherosclerosis is an inflammatory disease. *Am Heart J* 138: S419–420
111 Niwa S, Totsuka T, Hayashi S (1996) Inhibitory effect of fluvastatin, an HMG-CoA reductase inhibitor, on the expression of adhesion molecules on human monocyte cell line. *Int J Immunopharmacol* 18: 669–675
112 Lefer AM, Campbell B, Shin YK, Scalia R, Hayward R, Lefer DJ (1999) Simvastatin preserves the ischemic-reperfused myocardium in normocholesterolemic rat hearts. *Circulation* 100: 178–184
113 Scalia R, Gooszen ME, Jones SP, Hoffmeyer M, Rimmer DM, 3rd, Trocha SD, Huang PL, Smith MB, Lefer AM, Lefer DJ (2001) Simvastatin exerts both anti-inflammatory and cardioprotective effects in apolipoprotein e-deficient mice. *Circulation* 103: 2598–2603
114 Stalker TJ, Lefer AM, Scalia R (2001) A new HMG-CoA reductase inhibitor, rosuvastatin, exerts anti- inflammatory effects on the microvascular endothelium: the role of mevalonic acid. *Br J Pharmacol* 133: 406–412
115 Ridker PM, Rifai N, Clearfield M, Downs JR, Weis SE, Miles JS, Gotto AM Jr (2001) Measurement of C-reactive protein for the targeting of statin therapy in the primary prevention of acute coronary events. *N Engl J Med* 344: 1959–1965
116 Baumann H, Gauldie J (1994) The acute phase response. *Immunol Today* 15: 74–80
117 Koenig W, Sund M, Frohlich M, Fischer HG, Lowel H, Doring A, Hutchinson WL, Pepys MB (1999) C-Reactive protein, a sensitive marker of inflammation, predicts future risk of coronary heart disease in initially healthy middle-aged men: results from the MONICA (Monitoring Trends and Determinants in Cardiovascular Disease) Augsburg Cohort Study, 1984 to 1992. *Circulation* 99: 237–242
118 Ridker PM, Cushman M, Stampfer MJ, Tracy RP, Hennekens CH (1997) Inflammation, aspirin,

and the risk of cardiovascular disease in apparently healthy men. *N Engl J Med* 336: 973–979
119 Ridker PM, Buring JE, Shih J, Matias M, Hennekens CH (1998) Prospective study of C-reactive protein and the risk of future cardiovascular events among apparently healthy women. *Circulation* 98: 731–733
120 Ridker PM, Hennekens CH, Buring JE, Rifai N (2000) C-reactive protein and other markers of inflammation in the prediction of cardiovascular disease in women. *N Engl J Med* 342: 836–843
121 Liuzzo G, Biasucci LM, Gallimore JR, Grillo RL, Rebuzzi AG, Pepys MB, Maseri A (1994) The prognostic value of C-reactive protein and serum amyloid a protein in severe unstable angina. *N Engl J Med* 331: 417–424
122 Mendall MA, Patel P, Ballam L, Strachan D, Northfield TC (1996) C-reactive protein and its relation to cardiovascular risk factors: a population-based cross-sectional study. *BMJ* 312: 1061–1065
123 Bhakdi S, Torzewski M, Klouche M, Hemmes M (1999) Complement and atherogenesis: binding of CRP to degraded, nonoxidized LDL enhances complement activation. *Arterioscler Thromb Vasc Biol* 19: 2348–2354
124 Zhang YX, Cliff WJ, Schoefl GI, Higgins G (1999) Coronary C-reactive protein distribution: its relation to development of atherosclerosis. *Atherosclerosis* 145: 375–379
125 Torzewski J, Bowyer DE, Waltenberger J, Fitzsimmons C (1997) Processes in atherogenesis: complement activation. *Atherosclerosis* 132: 131–138
126 Musial J, Undas A, Gajewski P, Jankowski M, Sydor W, Szczeklik A (2001) Anti-inflammatory effects of simvastatin in subjects with hypercholesterolemia. *Int J Cardiol* 77: 247–253
127 Ridker PM, Rifai N, Lowenthal SP (2001) Rapid reduction in C-reactive protein with cerivastatin among 785 patients with primary hypercholesterolemia. *Circulation* 103: 1191–1193
128 Ridker PM, Rifai N, Pfeffer MA, Sacks F, Braunwald E (1999) Long-term effects of pravastatin on plasma concentration of C-reactive protein. The Cholesterol and Recurrent Events (CARE) Investigators. *Circulation* 100: 230–235
129 Ridker PM, Rifai N, Pfeffer MA, Sacks FM, Moye LA, Goldman S, Flaker GC, Braunwald E (1998) Inflammation, pravastatin, and the risk of coronary events after myocardial infarction in patients with average cholesterol levels. Cholesterol and Recurrent Events (CARE) Investigators. *Circulation* 98: 839–844
130 Albert MA, Staggers J, Chew P, Ridker PM (2001) The pravastatin inflammation CRP evaluation (PRINCE): rationale and design. *Am Heart J* 141: 893–898
131 Crouse JR, Byington RP, Furberg CD (1998) HMG-CoA reductase inhibitor therapy and stroke risk reduction: an analysis of clinical trials data. *Atherosclerosis* 138: 11–24
132 Dalkara T, Yoshida T, Irikura K, Moskowitz MA (1994) Dual role of nitric oxide in focal cerebral ischemia. *Neuropharmacology* 33: 1447–1452
133 Huang PL, Huang Z, Mashimo H, Bloch KD, Moskowitz MA, Bevan JA, Fishman MC (1995) *Hypertension* in mice lacking the gene for endothelial nitric oxide synthase. *Nature* 377: 239–242
134 Huang Z, Huang PL, Ma J, Meng W, Ayata C, Fishman MC, Moskowitz MA (1996) Enlarged infarcts in endothelial nitric oxide synthase knockout mice are attenuated by nitro-L-arginine. *J Cereb Blood Flow Metab* 16: 981–987
135 Endres M, Laufs U, Huang Z, Nakamura T, Huang P, Moskowitz MA, Liao JK (1998) Stroke protection by 3-hydroxy-3-methylglutaryl (HMG)-CoA reductase inhibitors mediated by endothelial nitric oxide synthase. *Proc Natl Acad Sci USA* 95: 8880–8885
136 Lefer AM, Scalia R, Lefer DJ (2001) Vascular effects of HMG CoA-reductase inhibitors (statins) unrelated to cholesterol lowering: new concepts for cardiovascular disease. *Cardiovasc Res* 49: 281–287

HMG-CoA Reductase Inhibitors
ed. by G. Schmitz and M. Torzewski

Indications and contra-indications for statin treatment (primary and secondary prevention of hypercholesterolemia)

Hans-P. Thomas and Elisabeth Steinhagen-Thiessen

Charité, Medical Faculty of Humboldt University of Berlin, Virchow-Clinic, Medizinische Poliklinik, LDL-Apherese, Mittelallee 11, D-13353 Berlin, Germany

Introduction

Cardiovascular diseases continue to be the most common cause of death in western countries. Along with mortality, morbidity following a myocardial infarction or stroke is of particular relevance, because, in addition to the considerable impairment to health, it creates immense economic demands. Atherosclerosis plays a central role as an etiological component in the development of this disease. The scientific data published in the past decade are as diverse as atherosclerosis as a multifactorial occurrence is complex. Epidemiological studies clearly showed that there is a replicable and independent relationship between the total cholesterol (TC) levels and the incidence of coronary heart disease (CHD). The significance of cholesterol for the development of CHD had become clear even in the 1980s [1]. This relationship stretches over a wide range of cholesterol levels and includes patients with normal or only slightly elevated levels [2, 3]. Primary diseases of the lipid metabolism are the most common hereditary diseases in adults with 1:200 (familial combined hyperlipidemia) to 1:500 (familial hypercholesterolemia) people affected in the population, and are accompanied by a very high risk of developing a symptomatic coronary disease before the age of 50. Cross-sectional studies reveal disorders of the lipid metabolism in as much as 40–50% of the population.

This means that cholesterol can be regarded as the outstanding and causal risk factor, since there is a strong and consistent relationship between the level of cholesterol and CHD, and this is based on a plausible pathophysiological mechanism. Moreover, the treatment of lipid disorders has proved to be highly effective in a series of studies [4–8]. It was shown that atherosclerosis, as the foundation of cardiovascular diseases, can be delayed and that the risk of further cardiovascular events in patients who have already suffered a myocardial infarction or stroke can be reduced effectively. In these studies, HMG-

CoA reductase inhibitors (statins) were employed for lipid lowering. Statins are a group of substances that have proved very effective and with high tolerability. The successes obtained using these drugs have not only been achieved for patients with hypercholesterolemia, but also for people with average cholesterol levels and these successes can also be obtained in the presence of other risk factors such as smoking, hypertension and diabetes.

Nevertheless, even today, disorders in the lipid metabolism are often only diagnosed when end points such as myocardial infarction and stroke have occurred. Furthermore, only approximately 32% of coronary patients in secondary prevention are treated with lipid-lowering drugs [9], although with regard to CHD therapy, for example, statins are now well established as a standard therapy along with acetylsalicylic acid and beta-blockers. At the moment there are no population-based strategies for comprehensive implementation of diagnosis and treatment guidelines to deal with this situation effectively. And yet the area of lipids offers us the opportunity of acting preventively to avert or at least delay cardiovascular events.

The mechanism of atherosclerosis

Atherosclerosis is remarkable for its complex etiology and is influenced in various ways by the presence of risk factors. Lipoproteins, which are deposited on the arterial wall, play a central role in the pathogenesis. Almost all lipoproteins are involved in this process. LDL cholesterol in its small dense form is considered to be especially atherogenic [10]. In addition, decisive, atherogenesis-promoting characteristics are attributed to very low-density lipoprotein (VLDL), remnant lipoproteins [11] and lipoprotein(a) [12]. An exception to this canon is high-density lipoprotein (HDL), which is able to mobilize cholesterol from the artery wall and transport it from there to the liver [13].

An increase in serum concentrations of lipids can lead to a pathological thickening of the arterial wall. This is characterized by intra- and extracellular lipid storage as well as by an accumulation of foam cells, which originate from monocytes or vascular muscle cells. The end point of this development is when the plaque ruptures and the lipid-rich core washes out into the bloodstream to cause the occlusion of an arterial vessel.

Indications for treatment in secondary prevention

In the last few years, the treatment of lipid disorders has proved to be extraordinarily effective in patients where CHD has already manifested itself. This is primarily the case where patients have elevated cholesterol levels. Since mortality rises by up to 10 times in CHD patients, consistent treatment strategies are needed, because it is no longer a case of statistical risk, but a resultant disease that requires therapy.

The following section contains a closer examination of the studies involving statins in order that evidence-based treatment strategies may be determined. Common to all the studies is the fact that both the treated group and the placebo group were given repeated and detailed instruction about dietary measures.

The Scandinavian Simvastatin Survival Study (4S) [7] can be considered a milestone among the investigations into the impact of cholesterol lowering on the mortality and morbidity of patients with CHD. 4444 patients with angina or previously suffered myocardial infarction with a serum cholesterol level of 212–309 mg/dl (5.5–8.0 mmol/l) were randomized for a double-blind therapy with simvastatin (20 or 40 mg) or placebo. The end points of the study were defined as overall mortality, serious CHD events (CHD-related death and non-fatal myocardial infarction), other acute atherosclerotic events, and myocardial revascularization procedures.

As expected, the treatment group showed a lowering of the TC and LDL cholesterol (–26% and –36%) as well as a rise in HDL cholesterol (+7%). However, the outstanding finding of the 5.4 year study period was the highly significant reduction in the risk of mortality and morbidity in the simvastatin group. Overall mortality was reduced by 31% (182 deaths in the simvastatin group *vs* 256 deaths in the placebo group), while coronary mortality fell by even more (–43%). The superiority of statin medication was also demonstrated in the secondary end points. The relative risk of a serious coronary event (cardiac death, non-fatal myocardial infarction or resuscitation following cardiac arrest) was 0.66. Simvastatin also made it less likely that a patient would have to undergo an aortocoronary bypass operation or angioplasty. The relative risk for that was 0.66. For the first time, it was possible to demonstrate that this effect was not gender-specific and that it included patients over 60. Although the effect was not as pronounced for the latter, it was still significant. The effects of the treatment increased with the length of the therapy and were first able to be detected after about a year. The risk of coronary death and non-fatal myocardial infarction declined by 26% in the first two years and even by 46% after that. This effect was achieved whether or not the patients smoked or suffered from hypertension.

The study also confirmed that there is no increase in non-cardiovascular causes of death as a result of cholesterol lowering. The number of violent deaths and fatal cancers, which were postulated in other survey articles about cholesterol-lowering studies [14, 15], were similar for both groups, and this in spite of the fact that the LDL cholesterol lowering was far stronger than in earlier studies.

4S is the first study in which a clear improvement in survival rates could be shown to result from cholesterol lowering by means of medication, and in that it is not alone.

Apart from 4S, there is the Cholesterol and Recurrent Events (CARE) study [6], the second large controlled study of lipid lowering using statins in CHD patients. It compared the benefits of lipid lowering obtained from pravastatin or placebo in patients with previously suffered myocardial infarction who exhibited a mean cholesterol level of less than 240 mg/dl (6.2 mmol/l) (mean value: 209 mg/dl) and a LDL cholesterol level of between 120 and 180 mg/dl (3.0–4.5 mmol/l) (mean value: 139 mg/dl). In the group given pravastatin, the TC and the LDL cholesterol were lowered significantly, by 20% and 28% respectively. HDL rose by an average 5%. Treatment with pravastatin resulted in the number of cardiac deaths as well as myocardial infarction falling by 20% and 24% respectively. The mean LDL level across a treatment period of five years could even be used to predict the rate of coronary events ($p = 0.007$), without it being possible, however, to show a linear relationship. Interestingly, however, there was no significant relationship between the extent of LDL lowering and the occurrence of cardiovascular events – either as an absolute reduction ($p = 0.97$), or as a percentage reduction ($p = 0.76$). The rate of cardiovascular events was positively affected by the lowering of the LDL level during the period of observation, if LDL cholesterol was lowered to a range between 174 and about 125 mg/dl. Further lowering of the LDL cholesterol produced no additional effect. A multivariate analysis of the triglycerides showed a weak but significant link to the occurrence of cardiovascular events. However, a connection between the level of HDL cholesterol and cardiovascular events could not be shown in the CARE study.

Unlike CARE and 4S, the intention of the LIPID study [16] was to examine the benefit of statins for patients with unstable angina by means of a controlled trial. More than 9,000 patients with an acute coronary syndrome were included, of whom 3,260 had unstable angina and 5,754 had previously suffered myocardial infarction. The cholesterol serum level was 155–270 mg/dl (4–7 mmol/l). The treatment group received pravastatin in a daily dosage of 40 mg. As a result of pravastatin, TC was reduced by 18%, LDL cholesterol by 25% and triglycerides by 12% while HDL cholesterol was raised by 6%. In findings similar to those of the CARE study, cardiovascular mortality was reduced by 24%, the rate of myocardial infarction by 28%, and revascularizations by 20%. In contrast to the CARE study, there was also a significant reduction in overall mortality, which could also be seen at a similar level in patients following myocardial infarction. The results were comparable to those of the 4S study in that they were not dependent on the initial lipid level and had no lower threshold.

The studies on secondary prevention have, therefore, made it clear that lipid-lowering medication is of great benefit to patients with CHD and contributes decisively to the reduction of cardiovascular events (Tab. 1). In addition to mortality, morbidity, with its immense medical, social and economic consequences, is obviously also affected favorably and the long-term prognosis of affected patients improved. In the 4S study, patients benefited who had elevated TC and LDL cholesterol, and in the LIPID study so did patients with average cholesterol levels (Fig. 1). Only the CARE study described a lower initial threshold, for which medication-induced lowering produced no clinical effect. No threshold was observed in the 4S study and the much larger LIPID

Table 1. Characteristics and outcome of 3 controlled cholesterol-lowering trials using statin drugs

Characteristics	4S[1] (1994)	CARE[2] (1996)	LIPID[3] (1998)
No. of participants	4444	4159	9014
Follow-up, mean (years)	5,4	5,0	6,1
Study drug	Simvastatin	Pravastatin	Pravastatin
Baseline data			
Age, mean (years)	59	59	62
Age > 64 years (%)	23	31	39
Women (%)	19	14	17
History of myocardial infarction (%)	79	100	64
Cholesterol level, mean (mg/dl & mmol/l)			
Total cholesterol	260 (6.75)	209 (5.40)	218 (5.64)
LDL-cholesterol	188 (4.87)	139 (3.59)	150 (3.88)
HDL-cholesterol	46 (1.19)	39 (1.01)	36 (0.93)
Triglycerides	58 (1.50)	67 (1.76)	61 (1.58)
Net change in lipid levels, mean (%)			
Total cholesterol	–26	–20	–18
LDL-cholesterol	–36	–28	–25
HDL-cholesterol	+7	+5	+5
Triglycerides	–17	–14	–11
Proportional risk reduction (%) (95% confidence intervall)			
Major coronary events	31 (26 to 36)	25 (10 to 38)	29 (20 to 36)
Coronary deaths	43 (38 to 55)	20 (–5 to 39)	25 (12 to 36)
Cardiovascular deaths	36 (20 to 49)	15 (–11 to 34)	32 (–25 to 63)
Noncardiovascular deaths	6 (–41 to 38)	–3 (–45 to 27)	17 (–2 to 33)
All-cause deaths	31 (16 to 44)	9 (–12 to 36)	24 (14 to 33)

[1] 4S indicates Scandinavian Simvastatin Survival Study;
[2] CARE, Cholesterol and Recurrent Events trial;
[3] LIPID, Long-term Intervention with Pravastatin in Ischaemic Disease trial.

study. The existence of such a threshold cannot be explained in terms of pathophysiology, either. On the other hand, the expected therapy effects are smaller, the lower the initial LDL level. Based on the data available, the National Cholesterol Education Program (NCEP) [17] recommends using drugs for secondary prevention to lower LDL cholesterol from an initial value of 130 mg/dl or above. The WOSCOPS data, according to which, lowering LDL cholesterol by 25% is sufficient for an optimal treatment effect, were not backed up in the 4S and LIPID studies. Both studies showed the clinical effect to be greater, the more LDL cholesterol was lowered. In the 4S study, a lowering of the LDL cholesterol level by 1% caused a 1.7% reduction in the incidence of coronary events. The logical consequence of these findings, to lower LDL cholesterol as much as possible, is also backed up by the results from the Post CABG study [18], where the patients benefited from an aggressive LDL reduction to under 100 mg/dl (2.6 mmol/l). The NCEP currently recommends using drugs in secondary prevention to lower LDL cholesterol to under

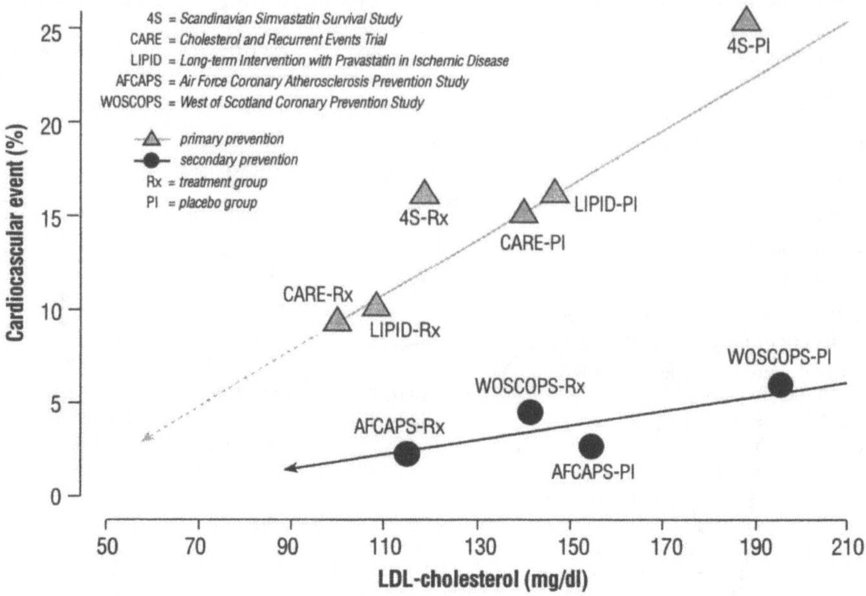

Figure 1. Relationship between the reduction of LDL-cholesterol and the frequency of major cardiovascular events in primary and secondary prevention trials.

100 mg/dl (2.6 mmol/l). Studies have shown that these are realistic targets, that can even be achieved at the family doctor's practice [19]. Moreover, it can be assumed that these patients will benefit from the secondary effects of this class of substances, such as fibrinogen lowering, reduced blood viscosity or activation of endothelial NO synthase [20]. It is clear from the data in the LIPID study that the lipid levels of patients with unstable angina should be checked immediately after the acute episode, and, if necessary, statin therapy should be initiated. In this way, there is a better chance of decisively improving the prognosis of the patient.

Unfortunately, there are still major problems with practical implementation on a day-to-day basis. At present, for example, only one in three coronary patients is treated with lipid-lowering drugs [9], although the guidelines in the USA [17] and Europe [21] have been providing clear recommendations for many years. There is a discrepancy between theory and practice in the treatment of diabetics, a group of patients with high coronary risk. There has also been a lack of success in putting study findings into practice for older patients who have a worse prognosis where CHD is present and following acute myocardial infarction.

What, however, is the situation for patients whose complaints mean that they have been advised to have invasive cardiac treatment? This question was the subject of the AVERT study [22]. The study was designed to test the clinical benefit of aggressive lipid lowering in patients scheduled for immediate angioplasty. In the course of this study, 341 patients suffering from mild to moderate anginal complaints or significant stenosis of one or two coronary arteries were divided into two treatment groups and thus subjected to an unprecedented comparison of two very different treatment strategies. All the patients had coronary sclerosis with at least 50% stenosis of a main artery. In the course of the study a random selection of the patients actually underwent angioplasty while the rest received 80 mg atorvastatin per day. In the PTCA group, in which the patients received a conventional therapy (including lipid-lowering medication) after the angioplasty, the LDL cholesterol was lowered to a mean level of 119 mg/dl (about 18 per cent). In the group treated with 80 mg atorvastatin, the effect of the lipid lowering on the LDL cholesterol was much more pronounced at –46 per cent, so that a mean LDL level of 77 mg/dl was able to be achieved. After 18 months, it could be seen that the rate of ischemia-related complications in the atorvastatin group was lower than in the patient group treated with PTCA. As in the 4S and Post CABG studies, the aggressively treated group was able to show – but only with a trend towards statistical significance in this case – a reduction (–36%) in revascularization procedures. The period before the occurrence of ischemic events was significantly longer in the statin group than following angioplasty. A reduction in angina symptoms was also achieved. However, a slight advantage was recorded for PTCA with regard to anginal symptoms.

Statins are credited with having other effects as well as cholesterol lowering. For example, experimental data for fluvastatin suggest that this substance inhibits the proliferation and migration of smooth muscle cells. This hypothesis served as the starting point of a study [23] which investigated the rate of restenosis after balloon angioplasty. These restenoses are not the result of new cholesterol deposition, but are attributed to an excess proliferation of arterial muscle cells. The study looked at 1054 patients who required balloon angioplasty due to significant coronary stenosis. Treatment with fluvastatin 80 mg/day or placebo was initiated two weeks before the surgery and maintained until the control angiography around six months later. The primary end point was the mean luminal diameter. The clinical end points were defined as death, myocardial infarction, surgical revascularization or angioplasty. As expected, there was a reduction of TC by 24% and LDL cholesterol by 33% in the treatment group. The hypothesis of there being an effect on the rate of restenosis could not, however, be substantiated by this study. The angiographic changes were similar in the two groups. However, there was a difference regarding clinical end points. There were 17 deaths or myocardial infarctions in the placebo group, whereas there were only 6 in the treatment group.

Statins seem to be capable of delaying the moment when angioplasty is needed. But on no account can a drug treatment replace a PTCA if patients develop anginal complaints at the slightest physical exertion. The idea of being able to affect restenosis after PTCA by pharmacological means was not backed up by the study.

Indications for statin treatment in primary prevention

Because of the high rates of cardiovascular disease, great significance must also be attached to primary prevention. However, in an era of constantly rising expenditure on health care, drug therapies should only be carried out – especially in the case of healthy individuals – if a substantial benefit to health is the result. On this topic, therefore, the question needs to be answered as to whether the rates of cardiovascular events and mortality can be lowered by means of cholesterol lowering, and as to which patients require treatment. In the pre-statin era, the need for a primary preventive therapy tended to be regarded with critical scepticism. In the LRC and Helsinki Heart Study [24, 25], while a reduction in cardiac events was able to be obtained as a result of cholesterol lowering, overall mortality was not able to be affected positively. Insufficient cholesterol lowering was discussed as a possible reason for this.

In contrast to these early studies, the WOSCOPS study [8] investigated the influence of an effective lipid-lowering therapy with pravastatin on the event rate of non-fatal myocardial infarction and cardiovascular mortality in men with hypercholesterolemia but no CHD. Given the high number of participants (6595), a statistically significant decrease in clinical events could be aimed for. With the population sample studied (men aged 45 to 64 with an average TC of 272 ± 23 mg/dl (7 mmol ± 0.69 mmol/l)), a significant reduction in clinical cardiovascular events was achieved in the 4.9-year follow-up period as a result of giving 40 mg pravastatin compared to the placebo. Lowering the total cholesterol by 20% (LDL cholesterol by 26%) resulted in a 31% fall in coronary events being observed. Non-fatal myocardial infarctions fell by 31% and cardiovascular deaths by 32%. Overall mortality was reduced by 22% (marginally significant: $p = 0.051$). This study was the first primary preventive study to achieve a reduction in clinical cardiovascular events with a marginally significant reduction of overall mortality by means of lipid-lowering drugs. Of additional interest was the observation, also made in secondary prevention studies, that the event curves began to diverge at an early stage – in this study after only six months. The use of pravastatin to lower cholesterol in men with hypercholesterolemia in primary prevention led to a reduction of clinical events without any increased risk in other areas. Of course, limitations in the data analysis are primarily the result of the study's chosen sample group. Because the WOSCOPS study was limited to middle-aged males, it investigated a population with an above-average risk of cardiovascular disease. Women were not included because of their lower incidence of cardiovascular events [26]. With the average age being 55 and no patient over 65, the significance of the data for older persons is unclear. Beyond that, the criticism can also be leveled that the study was performed in one country only and that there was no consideration of different morbidity data in other European countries.

In the AFCAPS/TexCAPS study [4], a comparative study was made between lovastatin and a placebo on the primary prevention of a first acute coronary event (angina, myocardial infarction, angioplasty, or bypass operation) in women and men with average cholesterol values. 5608 men and 997 women aged between 45 and 73 were randomly distributed among the study group and the control group. The study group received 20–40 mg lovastatin per day. The mean TC concentrations were 221 mg/dl (5.71 mmol/l), the LDL cholesterol averaged 150 mg/dl (3.89 mmol/l), the HDL cholesterol 36 mg/dl (0.94 mmol/l) and 40 mg/dl (1.03 mmol/l) for women. The average triglyceride concentrations were 158 mg/dl (1.78 mmol/l), and the follow-up observation period lasted 5.2 years.

In the treatment group, a 25% lowering of LDL cholesterol was achieved, while HDL was raised by 6%. The use of lovastatin meant that the incidence of a first acute cardiac event was able to be reduced by 36%. The relative risk of an acute myocardial infarction was 0.60, or 0.68 for angina, or 0.67 for revascularization surgery. It was therefore possible to reduce cardiac events by 38%. The results applied to both men and women. The study made it clear that a daily dose of 20–40 mg lovastatin – especially in combination with a balanced diet, physical exercise and a reduction in the known risk factors for cardiovascular conditions (smoking, excess weight, etc.) – is very suitable for reducing the cardiovascular risk in healthy men over 45 and women over 55 with HDL below 50 mg/dl or LDL levels above 130 mg/dl, even in a population with a very low risk of cardiovascular diseases. Analysis of the sub-groups clearly showed that participants with high blood pressure and diabetes benefited from lovastatin medication especially, exhibiting a 43% reduction in the risk of cardiovascular events in each case. The risk of a cardiac event in women was reduced even further by 54%. Similarly to the West of Scotland Coronary Prevention Study, the effects were evident after only 12 months. No threshold could be observed on the benefit gained from cholesterol lowering. This was also what was new about the study, in that compared to previous trials with cholesterol-lowering drugs, the effects of such a therapy were studied on patients who exhibited average levels for TC and LDL cholesterol but below-average HDL cholesterol (described by lipid percentiles of a cohort of the National Health and Nutrition Examination Survey [27] balanced for age and sex with no cardiovascular disease).

This study makes it clear, once again, that HDL cholesterol should also be included in the assessment of cardiovascular risk. This finding is supported by epidemiological studies such as the Framingham Heart Study [28] and the PROCAM study [29], which were able to point to an inverse relationship between the level of HDL cholesterol and the risk of CHD (Fig. 2). This relationship is independent of gender. Even a rise in HDL by 1 mg/dl was associated with a reduction in the risk of CHD of 2% in men and 3% in women. This means that even small changes in HDL produce a considerable effect on the clinical outcome parameters. In addition, treatment with lovastatin provides a therapeutic option for patients with low HDL levels.

In primary prevention, identifying those who are at risk is the first step leading to a rational system of prevention. Prevention has the aim of not allowing complaints and diseases to arise in the first place. The World Health

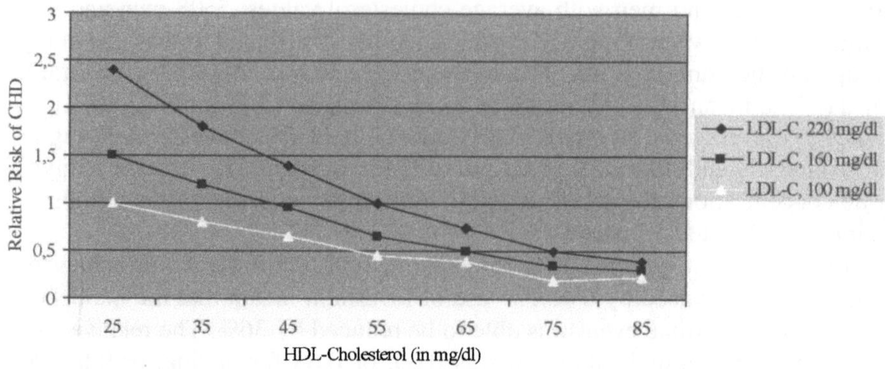

Figure 2. Relationship of HDL-C and LDL-C levels on relative risk of CHD in the Framingham Heart Study. (Adapted from [28]).

Organization (WHO) has subdivided the term prevention: primary prevention is used to describe measures that contribute to maintaining the health of the perfectly healthy and avoiding the development of diseases in them. Risk factors identify the factors that are statistically connected with certain diseases. These can favor the initial development of a disease without having to be causally responsible for them. A distinction is made between primary risk factors (factors that are responsible for the initial development of a disease) and secondary risk factors (factors that cause a worsening of the disease). In addition, risk factors are summarized into three different groups:

1. Internal risk factors (which represent diseases already): for example, lipid disorders (e.g., elevated cholesterol levels), high blood pressure (hypertension), blood glucose (diabetes).
2. External risk factors (lifestyle and lifestyle-related risk factors): e.g., smoking, stress, lack of exercise, bad diet, excess weight.
3. Constitutional risk factors (inherent, unalterable risk factors): e.g., sex, age, race, blood group.

The dividing line between primary prevention and secondary prevention is fluid. Many patients are diagnosed after manifestation of CHD (e.g., myocardial infarction). Moreover, even cardiological diagnosis is normally only sensitive enough to recognize, for example, exertion-related myocardial ischemia using tread mill or stress echocardiography once coronary stenosis has become extreme. This means that there must be a not inconsiderable number of people who per definition are in secondary prevention but who may be assessed as being primary prevention cases. Furthermore, it has become clear that the level of LDL cholesterol by itself does not provide enough information about the necessity for treatment. From the data contained in the GRIPS study [12], it can be concluded that a LDL cholesterol level of 150–160 mg/dl (3.9–4.2 mmol/l) on its own without other risk factors does not represent an elevated coronary risk, but that this would be the case with levels of 200 mg/dl (5.2 mmol/l) or more. However, if other risk factors are added, then their effect is potentiated. It is therefore necessary to establish individual risk management programs for each individual patient. But which individuals actually require a therapy? The authors of the AFCAPS study [4] estimated that approximately 17% of the reference population are in need of treatment according to the recommendations laid down in the NCEP guidelines. This would mean that potentially over 6 million people in the USA would come into consideration for statin treatment. But this would no doubt be infeasible on economic grounds alone.

The European Society of Cardiology recommends a drug therapy as soon as the expected 10-year event rate reaches or surpasses 20%. This was the case for older men (over 55) in the WOSCOPS study, and also for smokers and people with two or more additional risk factors or with atherosclerotic diseases. Regrettably, to this day no common standard for a definitive indication for primary preventive treatment has been created, so that the decision about treatment is left to the discretion of the physician.

On the basis of the large epidemiological studies, decision aids have been created such as the Wilson algorithm, which is based on the data from the Framingham Heart Study [30], or the PROCAM algorithm which includes 9 variables [29]. Figure 3 illustrates the incidence of coronary events that can be expected within an 8-year study period in men between the ages of 40 and 65 (in quintiles). Overall, the highest quintile has a more than 40-fold increased

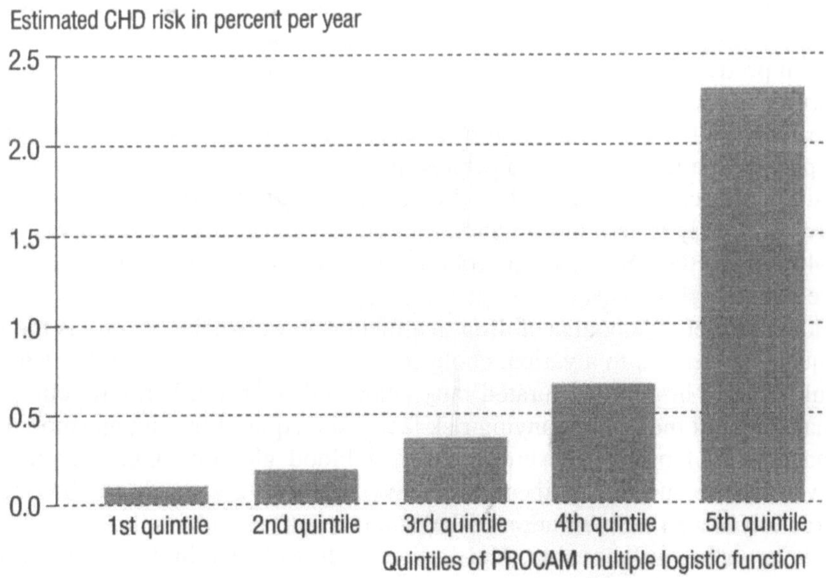

Figure 3.

risk. These methods make it possible to calculate an estimate of the individual risk of suffering a myocardial infarction. According to these algorithms, other risk factors should be present in addition to the elevated LDL cholesterol value of >170 mg/dl, before any decision is taken about statin treatment for primary prevention.

One recommendation oriented to the findings of epidemiological studies can also be taken from the principles established in the NCEP guidelines [31], as well as in national consensus discussions, for the threshold levels of total cholesterol and LDL cholesterol above which a diet or drug therapy should be introduced (Tab. 1). If there is a low coronary risk profile, i.e., no or only one risk factor for cardiovascular illnesses, then a LDL serum level of up to 155 mg/dl (4 mmol/l) is regarded as tolerable. A level of less than 135 mg/dl (3.5 mmol/l) should be the goal for individuals with two or more risk factors. On this basis then, statins should be employed if the desired levels cannot be obtained through a change in lifestyle. Where three risk factors are present, similar target levels to those for secondary prevention are now recommended, at least in Europe [32]. Another way to decide for or against statin treatment can be concluded from the data of the PROCAM study [29]. This showed that the risk of suffering a myocardial infarction grows exponentially with the ratio of LDL to HDL cholesterol. A quotient >4 is associated with a clear risk. While this quotient ignores other risk factors, it has nevertheless proved itself to be an adequate method of identifying patients in need of treatment.

Particular attention must also therefore be paid to HDL, since a low value is associated with an elevated coronary risk (Fig. 2). A number of studies were able to provide impressive evidence that HDL is an important "negative" risk factor for the development of CHD, which means that high HDL serum levels provide protection against atherosclerosis, and that raising this lipoprotein fraction produces positive effects on cardiovascular events [31]. Although the assertion is constantly made that endurance sport is the means of choice for increasing the HDL fraction, relatively excessive training sessions need to be completed on a regular basis to achieve measurable change in the HDL [33]. Statins could represent a potential alternative here. In the AFCAPS/TexCAPS study, as already stated, a 6% increase in HDL was obtained using lovastatin 20–40 mg. In the 4S study, the effects obtained with simvastatin were even more marked (HDL +8%).

However, before a course of drug treatment is initiated, the priority is for an adequate conversion to a varied, cholesterol-poor and fat-modified diet which should be rich in polyunsaturated fatty acids and fiber. Furthermore, optimal management of the accompanying risk factors is required (giving up smoking, management of blood pressure, control of blood glucose). Our experience shows that the success of these measures depends very much on thorough instruction as well as integration of the patient's partner and family, and a close physician-patient relationship. The earlier in life a change in diet takes place, the greater the probability is of long-term treatment success. If these measures are not enough, then drug therapy intervention must be discussed.

It is important to identify those who inherently carry a significantly elevated risk of CHD given the overwhelmingly dominant hereditary pattern of lipid disorders. An international WHO-supported project for familial hypercholesterolemia (MEDPED) [30] has been set up for patients. The purpose of MEDPED (Make Early Diagnosis – Prevent Early Deaths) is the early detection of affected family members of patients with familial hypercholesterolemia and confirmation of the familial form of the disease. To this end, all the family members are encouraged to undergo lipid screening. Following the final diagnosis, an individual therapy recommendation is discussed and agreed with the referring physicians for the patients and affected family members. Examining a patient's family results in the identification of on average 3–5 individuals who have a significantly elevated risk, due to the fact that hypercholesterolemia is an inherited autosomal dominant disorder with the consequence that 50% of family members are affected. The innovation of this approach is that one screening, in which simple, standardized, value-for-money methods are used, reveals a very high 'yield' of at-risk patients who are then accessible for lipid-lowering intervention. Such targeted screening is considerably superior to population screening. Due to the high level of involvement of patients and their family physicians, this strategy has proved extremely effective.

Stroke

Stroke has a high rate of incidence which increases steeply with age in the industrialized countries [34]. Although the risk factors are known, the incidence of ischemic stroke could not be significantly reduced either in Europe or the United States in the 1980s and 90s. Besides, current treatment for patients with established stroke is relatively ineffective with a high rate of permanent disability. These results contrast with the successes achieved in the fight against CHD. Given the increase of the elderly as a proportion of the population, a further increase in the disease can be expected with its many different consequences. An effective prevention of ischemic stroke would be of immense medical and economic importance for society.

New sub-group analyses show that not only patients with CHD benefit from lipid lowering, but that the incidence of stroke is also affected. Cerebrovascular events were able to be reduced by 28% in the 4S study, by 31% in the CARE study, and by 19% in the LIPID study.

The results of these studies are also significant because, according to existing epidemiological findings, hypercholesterolemia does not seem to play the dominant role as a risk factor in the etiology of stroke [35].

It is important in this regard to distinguish between ischemic strokes and those caused by hemorrhage. Patients with ischemic strokes seem to benefit the most from lipid lowering. In terms of pathophysiology, a decrease in the rate of progression of carotid atherosclerosis and plaque stabilization seem to be primarily responsible for this [36]. Conversely, there may be a negative association between serum cholesterol and hemorrhagic stroke.

In the 4S study [37], such cerebrovascular events fell by nearly 50%. The groups were easy to compare with regard to their stroke risk profiles. There were no indications of an increase in hemorrhagic strokes. Contrasted with the reduction in the risk of cardiac end points, it took 4 years for a visible advantage to appear for the treatment group with regard to strokes in the 4S study.

The CARE study [6] also investigated the frequency of strokes in order to test the potential effect of pravastatin on cerebrovascular events. A 32% reduction was achieved in apoplectic events. There was also a significant advantage for pravastatin if transient ischemic attacks (TIA) are added in, in that the number of all cerebrovascular events (stroke/TIA) was lowered from 124 to 92, representing a 27% reduction in risk.

The frequency of insult served as a secondary end point in the LIPID study [38] as well. While the results were less impressive than those for cardiac event reduction, the frequency of insult still fell by 19%. The question of whether this reduction in strokes for CHD patients also applies to older patients is the subject of the PROSPER study (Prospective Study of Pravastatin in the Elderly Risk). This placebo-controlled trial will test the hypothesis that tratment with pravastatin will diminish the risk of subsequent major vascular events in patients (70 to 82 years old) with pre-existing vascular disease.

But what of patients who have an increased risk of stroke, but who are formally designated for primary prevention? If one assumes that CHD patients with an increased risk of stroke are normally treated with statins, and that patients without CHD but at risk from stroke have probably not received any statins, then the significance of this question becomes clear. The studies on primary prevention published so far (WOSCOPS and AFCAPS) were not able to answer this question due to the chosen design with the sample population studied. Although WOSCOPS achieved a significant reduction of major coronary events in middle-aged men with hypercholesterolemia, there was no difference in the incidence of stroke between the treated and placebo groups [8]. A meta-analysis [39], which also studied the data from primary prevention trials, showed a 15% reduction in strokes in the patients treated with statins compared to the placebo group. However, this finding was not statistically significant. A large investigation into this question is currently being performed using cerivastatin, a statin of the third generation (RESPECT). The RESPECT study is being carried out on a cohort of elderly patients with high risk of stroke (high blood pressure, high cholesterol), because this group exhibits a high incidence of stroke and therefore seems most appropriate for the treatment. Patients with CHD or previous treatment with statins are not being included in the study. There is still some time to go before the first results provide information about whether patients, in particular older ones, can benefit from statin therapy and whether the standards of stroke treatment need modifying. Although a strict control of high cholesterol has not yet been sufficiently proved for primary prevention of stroke, it should be encouraged in patients with high risk of strokes because of benefits in terms of other diseases. In patients with CHD, statins clearly reduce the risk of stroke. The benefits of statin treatment in patients with previous stroke needs to be elucidated.

Diabetics

The positive effects of a statin therapy on women and the over–60 s with CHD have already been pointed out. But what is the case with diabetics, an example of a group with a particularly high risk of coronary events? Both type 1 and type 2 diabetes are associated with a marked increase in risk of CHD, cerebrovascular and peripheral vascular disease [10, 40, 41]. The relationship between diabetes and CHD is complex and plays out on a number of levels. Examples of what are considered to be particularly atherogenic factors include: an abnormal lipoprotein pattern and what is known as the lipid triad, i.e., high triglyceride levels; the presence of small dense LDL particles, which are classed as being especially atherogenic on account of their tendency to oxidize; and diminished HDL levels. In addition, there is often a coincidence between increased triglyceride concentrations and other factors of the metabolic syndrome (hypertension, insulin resistance, hyperuricemia). Recent studies have indicated that statin therapy could be a cornerstone of the pharmacological treatment in patients with diabetes. Although the use of fibrates also seems to be an appropriate solution for the lipoprotein pattern of diabetics, there is an indication for statin therapy in cases precisely where kidney function is limited or LDL cholesterol levels are >100 mg/dl (after a complete change in diet). This also makes sense with the atherogenic potency of oxidized LDL cholesterol levels, since these can be reduced effectively. Here again, information was able to be provided by means of a sub-group analysis of the 4S data [42]. 202 diabetics were compared with 4242 non-diabetic patients through analysis of sub-groups. Data from the 4S study can be used to work out an initial estimate of the effectiveness of a lipid-lowering therapy on diabetics. The changes to the lipoprotein profile of the diabetics resulting from treatment with simvastatin were comparable to those of the non-diabetics (total cholesterol –27%, LDL cholesterol –36%, HDL cholesterol +7% and triglycerides –11%). Serious CHD events were able to be reduced by 55% for this population group. In a widened 4S diabetes analysis, which took the diagnostic criteria of the American Diabetes Association (ADA) as its foundation, these positive effects were not only demonstrated for diabetics, but also for patients with impaired fasting glucose (IFG). Here, treatment with simvastatin led to a 38% drop in major coronary events. The benefits from the treatment could be even greater for diabetic CHD patients than for non-diabetic CHD patients.

Further studies investigating the benefit of a lipid-lowering therapy for diabetics are now underway (Heart Protection Study, ASPEN study, LDS study).

The old

The present demographic situation in the western industrialized countries is the result of various, longer-term processes. The general development is characterized by a steady rise in average life expectancy which has led to an increase in the percentage of over–60 s and exponential growth of those very advanced in years, meaning the over-eighties. Estimates show that this trend will become even more pronounced in the coming decades. The long uncertainty about whether dyslipidemia could be classed as a risk factor for the development and progression of CHD in old age was removed by large cohort studies [43–45]. Based on the data of a large U.S. trial, the assumption can be made that approximately 50% of people over 65 suffer from dyslipidemia [45]. The Framingham Heart Study [43] was also able to quantify elevated TC (>306 mg/dl; 0,94 mmol/l) as an independent risk factor for myocardial infarction and cardiovascular mortality in individuals over 65. A follow-up study confirmed this finding [44]. These data apply only up to the age of 70. There has only been sporadic emphasis on useful research into risk factors relating to advanced old age [46, 47]. An elevated level of cholesterol does not appear as important for the development of vascular processes in the oldest old as it does in younger patients. It can be assumed that the pattern of risk factors changes in old age, and that other factors (e.g., HDL cholesterol) become dominant influences.

So what effects does statin therapy have on older people? Although the 4S study was not designed for geriatric patients, analysis of sub-groups has been able to show the clear benefit of statin therapy for older patients [48]. Approximately 25% of the patients were aged between 65 and 70 when they began participating in the study. There was no less benefit from lipid lowering at this age than for younger patients. This applied to both the occurrence of cardiovascular events and overall mortality. Even in the 8-year intermediate analysis, no contrasting trend could be detected. The group treated with simvastatin exhibited a 34% reduction in overall mortality ($p = 0.009$) and a 43% reduction in cardiovascular mortality ($p = 0.003$). Thus, there is a substantially greater reduction in mortality and cardiovascular events in patients over 65 than in younger patients. The CARE study also showed a significant reduction in cardiovascular events in patients aged over 60 ($n = 2129$). Because the target level for LDL cholesterol in patients with CHD should be set at <100 mg/dl (2.6 mmol/l) and a change in diet alone is insufficient for this in many cases, statins are frequently indicated. Table 2 shows the results of prevention trials in the elderly.

How much of a benefit the therapy is for the very old remains pure speculation at the moment. Moreover, functional parameters have not been recorded in the studies available so far, even though they play a dominant role as a yardstick for success in geriatric patients. Hence, there is a considerable need for more research which seems to be urgently required in view of our society's changing age structure.

Table 2. Statins and the reduction of major coronary events in elderly patients: prevention studies

Characteristics	4S, 1997[1]	CARE, 1998[2]	LIPID, 1998[3]	AFCAPS, 1998[4]
Number of patients (Age/years)	1848 (>65)	1283 (60–75)	2168 (65–69) 1346 (>69)	1416 (>65)
Medication	Simvastatin	Pravastatin	Pravastatin	Lovastatin
Follow-up (years)	8	5	6,1	5,2
Risk reduction (in percent) (95% Confidenceinterval) Major coronary events	34 (16–48)	32 (15–46)	28 (11–41) 15 (8–33)	37 (31–50)

[1] 4S = Scandinavian Simvastatin Survival Study;
[2] CARE = Cholesterol and Recurrent Events trial;
[3] LIPID = Long-term Intervention With Pravastatin in Ischaemic Disease trial;
[4] AFCAPS = Air Force/Texas Coronary Atherosclerosis Prevention Study.

Contra-indications for statin therapy

The contra-indications for a statin therapy arise, on the one hand, from the spectrum of side effects or an oversensitivity to a constituent of this type of drug, and on the other, from areas of application where there has been insufficient study (e.g., on children) [49].

People who should be excluded from this treatment are those who suffer from an active liver disease or cholestasis or who exhibit a persistent elevation of liver enzymes. With statin therapy, rises in the liver function parameters are occasionally observed which are normally reversible and not a constraint on the therapy. Increases in liver enzymes up to 3 times the upper norm can generally be tolerated. Exceptionally, there may be clear and persistent increases in the serum transaminases, which force the therapy to be terminated. The gamma-glutamyl transferase, bilirubin and alkaline phosphatase can all increase as well [50]. Since these changes often occur at the start of the therapy, these parameters should be monitored somewhat more frequently at the beginning and then at 3–6 monthly intervals during the course of treatment.

Myopathies also represent a (relative) contra-indication for treatment with statins. Increases in creatine phosphokinase (CPK) are not unusual and are normally harmless [51]. The therapy must be broken off whenever any patient experiences diffuse muscular pains, muscle weakness and/or CPK increases, in order to stop the development of manifest myopathy. The simultaneous administration of immunosupressants (cyclosporine), fibrates or nicotinic acid derivatives also increases the likelihood of myopathies occurring [52]. However, rhabdomyolysis with secondary renal failure is observed only very rarely. Although hepatotoxicity and myotoxicity are rare, they occur more frequently where there is co-medication with preparations that are metabolized by means of cyclo-oxygenase P-450. Most of the statins are also metabolized in this way (simvastatin, atorvastatin, lovastatin, cerivastatin via P-450 3A4; fluvastatin via P-450 2C9). Only pravastatin is sulfatized, thus representing a therapeutic alternative. Lovastatin should not be administered together with nicotinic acid derivatives, since myopathy occurs in up to 1% of cases. No reduction in dose is necessary for patients with renal insufficiency, since there is only minor renal elimination of statins. Where kidney function is more severely restricted (creatinine clearance <30 ml/min.), decisions about higher doses should be carefully weighed up [53].

Peripheral neuropathy, sleep disorders and nightmares are all possibilities and can force the therapy to be abandoned [54]. For patients where central nervous side effects appear, a statin can be tried out which does not pass the blood-brain barrier (e.g., pravastatin) [50].

Statins are contra-indicated during pregnancy and breastfeeding. The reason for this is that cholesterol is an essential component for fetal development, including the synthesis of steroids and cell membranes.

On the whole, statin therapy is well tolerated. Side-effects are normally reversible and even with high dosages occur in fewer than 2% of patients [55].

Conclusion

Statins have become accepted as the therapy of choice in the management of hypercholesterolemia, mainly in patients with CHD. But even in primary prevention the use of statins makes it possible to lessen the risk of developing CHD.

With the statin therapies employed in the studies, TC was reduced on average by 20%, LDL cholesterol by 28% and triglycerides by 13%. HDL cholesterol rose by an average 5%. Under such therapy, the overall risk of cardiovascular events fell by 31%, and the risk of fatal coronary events by 29%. Cardiovascular mortality decreased by 27% and overall mortality was able to be reduced by 21%. The preparations employed were not associated with an increase in non-cardiovascular deaths in any of the studies. Nor was there any accumulation of malignant diseases in the treatment groups. These findings underline the significance of the application of statins in secondary prevention and, at the same time, show that a long-term therapy (over 5 years) lowers mortality and is well tolerated.

The optimal target for LDL cholesterol in secondary prevention is the subject of discussion. International consensus conferences have established a LDL target of <100 mg/dl (2.6 mmol/l) as the present upper limit. Patients who are unable to reach this target through a change in lifestyle have a clear indication for lipid-lowering drug therapy.

The positive effect of drug-induced lipid lowering was also proved in patients with only minor dyslipidemia or who were in primary prevention. However, a decision about drug intervention should be made on the basis of the patient's individual risk profile. Various algorithms are available for this purpose or else the recommendations of the NCEP guidelines can be referred to, for example.

The medication therapy effects of statins have been proved independent of gender and applicable up to the 75-year-old age group. There are insufficient data only for the very old (>75). Although limiting screening and therapy for such people is potentially dangerous, the applicability of data from intervention studies to elderly patients seems questionable. Further studies will have to be made to provide clarity about the treatment procedure in this age group.

Effective cholesterol reduction also has a beneficial influence on other atherosclerotic changes (stroke), although such resultant diseases have so far received much less attention in the literature. For patients with manifest atherosclerosis, an indication for treatment with statins seems to be supported by the data. The question of whether primary preventive intervention is appropriate can not yet be answered. Studies being carried out now will provide information on this just as they will for the treatment of elderly patients.

Contra-indications primarily concern hypersensitivity, active liver disease or unexplained persistent elevations of liver enzymes, muscle diseases, pregnancy and lactation. Other side-effects that would limit treatment employing a statin therapy are very rare. However, it must be noted that such preparations are not to be used during pregnancy and breastfeeding and that extending the treatment to children and the elderly must be examined critically.

If "Evidence-Based Medicine" (EBM) is taken as the guiding principle of medical practice, then the use of statins to lower cholesterol can surely serve as a perfect example of a sensible therapy approach. In order to help physicians provide a rational lipid-lowering treatment in line with EBM, therapy recommendations must be drawn up to serve as guidelines by appropriately qualified bodies. Such recommendations have been produced internationally for the area of lipid disorders. Only such guidelines drawn up according to EBM principles should be used as a basis for quality assurance in medicine. They impose procedural frameworks and thus protect against arbitrariness of treatment. If we succeed in applying these guidelines to daily practice, then a great many more patients will benefit, and a further reduction in morbidity and mortality from cardiovascular diseases will be the consequence. In the meantime, it has become more important to ensure that we actually put into practice what we know from numerous studies than to spend large amounts of time and money in a constant search for new treatments.

References

1 Stamler J, Wentworth D, Neaton JD, for the MRFIT Research Group (1986) Is the relationship between serum cholesterol and risk of premature death from coronary heart disease continuous and graded? Findings in 356,222 primary screenees of the Multiple Risk Factor Intervention Trial (MRFIT). *JAMA* 256: 2823–2828

2 Chen ZM, Peto R, Collins R, MacMahon S, Lu JR, Li WX (1991) Serum cholesterol concentration and coronary heart disease in population with low cholesterol concentrations. *BMJ* 303: 276–82

3 Levine GN, Keaney JF, Vita JA (1995) Cholesterol reduction in cardiovascular disease: clinical benefits and possible mechanisms. *N Engl J Med* 332: 512–521

4 Downs JR, Clearfield M, Weis S, Whitney E, Shapiro DR, Beere PA, Langendorfer A, Stein EA, Kruyer W, Gotto AM Jr (1998) Primary prevention of acute coronary events with lovastatin in men and women with average cholesterol levels: results of AFCAPS/TexCAPS. Air Force/Texas Coronary Atherosclerosis Prevention Study. *JAMA* 279: 1615–1622

5 Long Term Intervention with Pravastatin in Ischemic Disease (LIPID) Study Group (1998) Prevention of cardiovascular events and death with pravastatin in patients with coronary heart disease and a broad range of initial cholesterol levels. *N Engl J Med* 339: 1349–1357

6 Sacks FM, Pfeiffer MA, Moye LA, Rouleau JL, Rutherford JD, Cole TG, Brown L, Warnica JW, Arnold JMO, Wun CC et al, for the Cholesterol and Recurrent Event Trial Investigators (1996) The effect of pravastatin on recurrent coronary events after myocardial infarctions in patients with average cholesterol levels. *N Engl J Med* 335: 1001–1009

7 Scandinavian Simvastatin Survival Study Group (1994) Randomized trial of cholesterol lowering therapy in 4444 patients with coronary artery disease: the Scandinavian Simvastatin Survival Study (4S). *Lancet* 344: 1383–1389

8 Shepherd J, Cobbe SM, Ford I, Isles CG, Lorimer AR, MacFarlane PW, McKillop JH, Packard CJ (1995) Prevention of coronary artery disease with pravastatin in men with hypercholesterolemia. West of Scotland Coronary Prevention Study Group. *N Engl J Med* 333: 1303–1307

9 EUROASPIRE. A European Society of Cardiology survey of secondary prevention of coronary heart disease: principal results. EUROASPIRE Study Group (1997) European action on secondary prevention through intervention to reduce events. *Eur Heart J* 18: 1569–1582

10 Coresh J, Kwiterovich PO (1996) Small, dense low-density lipoprotein particles and coronary heart disease risk. A clear association with uncertain implications. *JAMA* 276: 914–915

11 Rapp JH, Lespine A, Hamilton RL, Colyvas N, Chaumeton AH, Tweedie-Hardman J, Kotite L, Kunitake ST, Havel RJ, Kane JP (1994) Triglyceride-rich proteins isolated by selected affinity anti-apolipoprotein B immunosorption from human atherosclerotic plaque. *Arterioscler Thromb* 14: 1767–1774

12 Cremer P, Nagel D, Labrot B, Mann H, Müller-Berninger R, Elster H, Seidel D (1997) Ten-year follow-up results from the Goettingen risk, incidence and prevalence study (GRIPS). I. Risk factors for myocardial infarction in a cohort of 5790 men. *Atherosclerosis* 129: 221–230

13 Oram F, Yokoyama S (1996) Apolipoprotein-mediated removal of cellular cholesterol and phospholipids. *J Lipid Res* 36: 2473–2491

14 Davey Smith G, Pekkanen J (1992) Should there be a moratorium on the use of cholesterol lowering drugs? *BMJ* 304: 431–434

15 Oliver MF (1991) Might treatment of hypercholesterolaemia increase non-cardiac mortality? *Lancet* 337: 1529–1531

16 Tonkin AM, for the LIPID Study Group (1995) Management of the Long-term Intervention with Pravastatin in Ischaemic Disease (LIPID): Study after the Scandinavian Sinvastatin Survival Study (4S). *Am J Cardiol* 76: 107c–112c

17 Expert panel on detection, evaluation, treatment of high blood cholesterol in adults (1993) Summary of the second report of the national cholesterol education program (NCEP). Expert panel on detection, evaluation and treatment of high blood cholesterol in adults (adult treatment panel II). *JAMA* 269: 3015–3023

18 The Post Coronary Artery Bypass Graft Trial Investigators (1997) The effect of aggressive lowering of low-density lipoprotein cholesterol levels, low-dose anticoagulation on obstructive changes in saphenous-vein coronary-artery bypass grafts. *N Engl J Med* 336: 153–162

19 Marz W, Wollschlager H, Klein G, Neiss A, Wehling M (1999) Safety of low-density lipoprotein cholestrol reduction with atorvastatin *versus* simvastatin in a coronary heart disease population (the TARGET TANGIBLE trial). *Am J Cardiol* 84: 7–13

20 Knopp RH (1999) Drug treatment of lipid disorders. *N Engl J Med* 341: 498–511

21 Pyorala K, De Backer G, Graham I, Poole-Wilson P, Wood D, on behalf of the task force (1994) Prevention of coronary heart disease in clinical practice. Recommendations of the task force of the European Society of Cardiology, European Atherosclerosis Society and European Society of Hypertension. *Eur Heart J* 15: 1300–1331

22 Pitt B, Waters D, Brown WV, van Boven AJ, Schwartz L, Title LM, Eisenberg D, Shurzinske L, McCormick LS (1999) Aggressive lipid-lowering therapy compared with angioplasty in stable coronary artery disease. Atorvastatin *versus* Revascularization Treatment Investigators. *N Engl J*

Med 341: 70–76
23 Serruys PW, Foley DP, Jackson G, Bonnier H, Macaya C, Vrolix M, Branzi A, Shepherd J, Suryapranata H, de Feyter PJ (1999) A randomized placebo-controlled trial of fluvastatin for prevention of restenosis after successful coronary balloon angioplasty; final results of the fluvastatin angiographic restenosis (FLARE) trial. *Eur Heart J* 20: 58–69
24 Strandberg TE, Salomaa VV, Naukkarinen VA, Vanhanen HT, Sarna SJ, Miettinen TA (1990) Long-term mortality after 5-year multifactorial primary prevention of cardiovascular diseases in middle-aged men. *JAMA* 266: 1225–1229
25 The Lipid Research Clinics Coronary Primary Prevention Trial results (1984) I. Reduction in incidence of coronary heart disease. *JAMA* 251: 351–364
26 Rich-Edwards J, Manson JE, Hennekens CH, Buring JE (1995) The primary prevention of coronary heart disease in women (medical progress). *N Engl J Med* 332: 1758–1766
27 Nation Center for Health Statistics (1996) Third National Health and Nutrition Examination Survey, 1988–1994, US NHANES III Examination Data File [CD-Rom]. Hyattsville, Md: Centers for Disease Control and Prevention. DHHS public use data file 76200
28 Kannel WB, Carter BL (1989) Initial drug therapy for hypertensive patients with hyperlipidemia. *Am Heart J* 118: 1012–1021
29 Assmann G, Schulte H, Cullen P (1997) New and classical risk factors – the Munster heart study (PROCAM). *Eur J Med Res* 2: 237–242
30 Williams RR, Hopkins PN, Stephenson S, Wu L, Hunt SC (1999) Primordial prevention of cardiovascular disease through applied genetics. *Prev Med* 29: S41-S49
31 The Expert Panel (1988) Report of the national cholesterol education program expert panel on detection evaluation, treatment of high blood cholesterol in adults. *Arch Intern Med* 148: 36–69
32 Wood D, De Backer G, Faergemann O, Graham I, Mancia G, Pyorala K (1998) Prevention of coronary heart disease in clinical practice: recommendations of the second joint task force of European and other societies for coronary prevention. *Atherosclerosis* 140: 199–270
33 Thompson PD, Cullinane EM, Sady SP, Flynn MM, Bernier DN, Kantor MA, Saritelli AL, Herbert PN (1988) Modest changes in high-density lipoprotein concentration and metabolism with prolonged exercise training. *Circulation* 78: 25–34
34 Wolf PA, D'Agostino RB, O'Neal MA, Sytkowski P, Kase CS, Belanger AJ, Kannel WB (1992) Secular trends in stroke incidence and mortality. The Framingham Study. *Stroke* 23: 1551–1555
35 Berger K, Schulte H, Stogbauer F, Assmann G (1998) Incidence and risk factors for stroke in an occupational cohort: the PROCAM Study. Prospective Cardiovascular Muenster Study. *Stroke* 29: 1562–1566
36 Salonen R, Nyyssonen K, Porkkala E, Rummukainen J, Belder R, Park JS, Salonen JT (1995) Kuopio Atherosclerosis Prevention Study (KAPS). A population-based primary preventive trial of the effect of LDL lowering on atherosclerotic progression in carotid and femoral arteries. *Circulation* 92: 1758–1764
37 Pedersen TR, Kjekshus J, Pyorala K, Olsson AG, Cook TJ, Musliner TA, Tobert JA, Haghfelt T (1998) Effect of simvastatin on ischemic signs, symptoms in the Scandinavian Simvastatin Survival Study (4S). *Am J Cardiol* 81: 333–355
38 White HD, Simes RJ, Anderson NE, Hankey G, Watson D, Hunt D, Colquhoun DM, Glasziou P, MacMahon S, Kirby AC et al (2000) Pravastatin therapy and the risk of stroke. *N Engl J Med* 343: 317–326
39 Crouse JR, Byington RP, Hoen HM, Furberg CD (1997) Reductase inhibitor monotherapy and stroke prevention. *Arch Intern Med* 157: 1305–1310
40 Haffner SM, Lehto S, Ronnemaa T, Pyorala K, Laakso M (1998) Mortality from coronary heart disease in subjects with type 2 diabetes, nondiabetic subjects with, without prior myocardial infarction. *N Engl J Med* 339: 229–234
41 Chun BY, Dobson AJ, Heller RF (1997) The impact of diabetes on survival among patients with first myocardial infarction. *Diabetes Care* 20: 704–708
42 Pyorala K, Pedersen TR, Kekshus J, Faergeman O, Olsson AG, Thorgeirsson G (1997) Cholesterol lowering with simvastatin improves prognosis of diabetic patients with coronary heart disease. A subgroup analysis of the Scandinavian Simvastatin Survival Study (4S). *Diabetes Care* 20: 614–620
43 Harris T, Cook EF, Kannel WB, Goldman L (1988) Proportional hazards analysis of risk factors for coronary heart disease in individuals aged 65 or older. The Framingham Heart Study. *J Am Geriatr Soc* 36: 1023–1028

44 Kronmal RA, Cain KC, Ye Z, Omenn GS (1993) Total serum cholesterol levels and mortality risk as a function of age. A report based on the Framingham data. *Arch Intern Med* 153: 1065–1067
45 Vital and health statistics (1994) National Hospital Discharge survey: Annual summary, Series 13: Data from the National Health Care Survey No. 128. *DHHS* Publication No. (PHS) 97-1789. Washington, D: US. Department of Health and Human Services, Center for Disease Control and Prevention, National Center for Health Statistics
46 Hillen T, Nieczaj R, Munzberg H, Schaub R, Borchelt M, Steinhagen-Thiessen E (2000) Carotid atherosclerosis, vascular risk profile and mortality in a population-based sample of functionally healthy elderly subjects: the Berlin ageing study. *J Intern Med* 247: 679–688
47 Steinhagen-Thiessen E, Borchelt M (1996) Morbidity, medication and functional limitations in very old age. *In*: KU Baltes, PB Meyer (eds):. *The Berlin Ageing Study*. Cambridge University Press, Cambridge, UK, 131–166
48 Miettinen TA, Pyorala K, Olsson AG, Musliner TA, Cook TJ, Faergeman O, Berg K, Pedersen T, Kjekshus J, for the Scandinavian Simvastatin Study Group (1997) Cholesterol-lowering therapy in women and elderly patients with myocardial infarction or angina pectoris. Findings from the Scandinavian Simvastatin Survival Study (4S). *Circulation* 96: 4211–4218
49 Duplaga BA (1999) Treatment of childhood hypercholesterolemia with HMG-CoA reductase inhibitors. *Ann Pharmacother* 33: 1224–1227
50 Beaird SL (2000) HMG-CoA reductase inhibitors: assessing differences in drug interactions and safety profiles. *J Am Pharm Assoc* 40: 637–644
51 Tikkanen MJ (1996) Statins: within-group comparisons, statin escape and combination therapy. *Curr Opin Lipidol* 7: 385–388
52 Ozdemir O, Boran M, Gokce V, Uzun Y, Kocak B, Korkmaz S (2000) A case with severe rhabdomyolysis and renal failure associated with cerivastatin-gemfibrozil combination therapy – a case report. *Angiology* 51: 695–697
53 Wheeler DC (1998) Statins and the kidney. *Curr Opin Nephrol Hypertens* 7: 579–584
54 Jeppesen U, Gaist D, Smith T, Sindrup SH (1999) Statins and peripheral neuropathy. *Eur J Clin Pharmacol* 54: 835–838
55 Ose L, Kastelein JJ, Scott R, Stein EA, Campodonico S, Escobar ID, Tate AC, Corsetti L, Shahane A, Mitchel YB et al for the WSEDP Research Group (1998) Efficacy and six-month safety of simvastatin 80 mg/day. Results from the worldwide simvastatin expanded dose program (WSEDP). *Nutr Metab Cardiovasc Dis* 8: 135–143

Clinical experience: studies with HMG-CoA reductase inhibitors

Helena K. Gylling[1] and Tatu A. Miettinen[2]

[1] *Department of Clinical Nutrition, University of Kuopio and Kuopio University Hospital, Kuopio, Finland*
[2] *Division of Internal Medicine, Department of Medicine, University of Helsinki, Helsinki, Finland*

Introduction

Before the hydroxy-methyl glutaryl CoA (HMG-CoA) reductase inhibitor (statin) era, it was known from animal experiments and from human angiographic studies that lowering of serum total and LDL cholesterol levels is followed by regression of atherosclerotic lesions in arteries [1]. It was also shown in humans that with extensive dietary and lifestyle changes it was possible to reduce the most important clinical outcome, coronary morbidity and mortality [2–5]. In addition, similar results were obtained with a couple of large-scale drug interventions with cholestyramine [6] and nicotinic acid [7]. On the basis of these studies, it could be anticipated that atherosclerosis is a reversible disease.

Since 1994, five large clinical trials of the beneficial effect of statins on coronary disease have been published [8–12]. These trials have revealed that extensive serum cholesterol reduction by HMG-CoA reductase inhibitors could actually be associated with a marked reduction in clinical manifestations of arterial atheromatosis, especially of myocardial infarction. The use of statins for cholesterol lowering has been dealt with in several extensive reviews, e.g., by refs [1], [13] and [14]. The present paper concentrates, first, on large clinical trials trying to figure out how effectively they prevent clinical manifestations of atheromatous disease in all arteries including not only coronary arteries, but also cerebral, carotic and peripheral arteries [15–17]. Second, effects of statins on serum non-cholesterol sterols and their clinical significance will be described.

Five large clinical statin trials

The five large trials [8–12] were double-blind, placebo-controlled interventions, including alltogether 30,817 subjects (Tab. 1). The Scandinavian Simvastatin Survival Study (4S), the Cholesterol and Recurrent Events

Table 1. Summary of five statin studies

Studies	Duration, years	Age, years	Sex	No of subjects	Serum lipids[a], mmol/l		Outcome		
					Serum cholesterol	LDL cholesterol	LDL cholesterol change %	Relative risk of MCE,%	Relative risk of total mortality, %
Secondary prevention									
4S [8] simvastatin 20–40 mg/d	5.4	35–70	F + M	4444	5.5–8.0 6.75	- 4.87	–35*	–34*	–30*
CARE [9] pravastatin 40 mg/d	5.0	21–75	F + M	4159	<6.2 5.40	3.0–4.5 3.59	–32*	–24*	–9, NS
LIPID [10] pravastatin 40 mg/d	6.1	31–75	F + M	9014	4.0–7.0 5.63	3.9 3.88	–25*	–24*	–22*
Primary prevention									
WOSCOPS [11] pravastatin 40 mg/d	4.9	45–64	M	6595	- 7.0	4.0–6.0 5.0	–26*	–31*	–22*
AFCAPS/TexCAPS [12] lovastatin 20–40 mg/d	5.2	45–73	F + M	6605	4.65–6.82 5.71	3.36–4.91 3.89	–25*	–25*	not determined

MCE = major coronary event. *$p < 0.05$ or less.
[a] first line: inclusion criteria, second line: mean of the study population.

(CARE) and the Long-term Intervention with Pravastatin in Ischaemic Disease (LIPID) trials were secondary prevention studies, whereas the West of Scotland Coronary Prevention Study (WOSCOPS) and the Air Force/Texas Coronary Atherosclerosis Prevention Study (AFCAPS/TexCAPS) were primary prevention studies. The duration varied from 5 to 6 years, and both LIPID and AFCAPS/TexCAPS were stopped earlier for efficacy. The age distribution varied from 21 to 75 years of age, and the number of women was 3916, constituting 13% of the study population.

The subjects in 4S and WOSCOPS were moderately hypercholesterolemic, whereas in the others they were only mildly hypercholesterolemic (Tab. 1). Low-normal HDL cholesterol level was also an inclusion criterion in AFCAPS/TexCAPS, and serum triglycerides were limited to <2.5 mmol/l in 4S, whereas in LIPID and AFCAPS/TexCAPS the levels were up to 5 mmol/l and 4.52 mmol/l, respectively.

None of the trials evaluated the efficacy of cholesterol lowering started immediately after an acute coronary attack on serum cholesterol concentration or on coronary events, even though CARE and LIPID were started at least 3 months after an acute event or coronary revascularization. The primary endpoint varied between the studies; in 4S it was total mortality, in CARE it was death from coronary heart disease or nonfatal acute myocardial infarction, in LIPID it was death from coronary heart disease, in WOSCOPS it was nonfatal myocardial infarction or death from coronary heart disease, and in AFCAPS/TexCAPS it was fatal or nonfatal myocardial infarction, unstable angina, or sudden cardiac death, respectively. For comparisons between the different trials, we have engaged major coronary event (MCE) as the outcome variable, which included death from coronary heart disease or nonfatal myocardial infarction in 4S, CARE, LIPID and WOSCOPS, whereas in AFCAPS/TexCAPS, unstable angina was also included.

Adverse events

In every trial, the number of adverse events was small, and statin was well tolerated. In 4S, 6% of those in both placebo and statin groups discontinued the study medication because of an adverse effect, and in CARE, the number of withdrawals in the statin group, 2.2% (45 subjects), was even significantly lower than in the placebo group (3.6%, 74 subjects). In the primary prevention trials, the number of withdrawals was larger, 13.8% in the lovastatin group and 13.8% in the placebo group in AFCAPS/TexCAPS and 29.6% and 30.8%, respectively, in WOSCOPS. The quality of adverse effects, including serious life-threatening episodes or diagnosis of any cancer, was identical in the placebo and statin groups in every study. However, the number of breast cancers was 12 in the pravastatin group vs 1 in the placebo group ($p = 0.002$) in CARE. The increment of liver transaminases that was more than 3 times and of creatine kinase that was greater than 10 times the upper normal limit was rare, and the incidence was similar in both statin and placebo groups, about 0.6% for both.

Changes in serum lipids

LDL cholesterol was significantly reduced from baseline values by 25%–35% (Tab. 1) corresponding to a reduction of approximately from –1 mmol/l to almost –2 mmol/l. The reduction was maintained during the whole study period [11, 18–20]. The achieved LDL cholesterol value varied from 2.5 mmol/l in CARE, 2.91 mmol/l in LIPID, 2.96 mmol/l in AFCAPS/TexCAPS, about 3 in 4S and to about 3.7 mmol/l in WOSCOPS, respectively. The findings indicate that the goal of LDL cholesterol, <2.6 mmol/l, was usually obtained in coronary patients in less than half of the participants.

In every study, HDL cholesterol was significantly increased from 5% to 8%, such that the LDL to HDL cholesterol ratio was significantly reduced by 28% from baseline [21]. Serum triglycerides were also significantly reduced in every study from 11% to 15%. The lipid changes were similar in men and women [12].

Total mortality

Death from all causes was lower in the statin vs placebo group such that the relative risk of total mortality was significantly reduced by 30% in 4S, and by 22% in LIPID and WOSCOPS (Tab. 1). For instance, in LIPID the number of deaths was 498 (11.0%) in the statin vs 633 (14.1%) in the placebo group, and in 4S, the respective figures were 182 (8.2%) vs 256 (11.5%). In the primary prevention trials, the figures were smaller. In CARE, 180 subjects in the statin and 196 in the placebo group died, but due to small numbers the risk reduction was not significant, and in AFCAPS/TexCAPS, the number of deaths was even smaller, 80 in the statin and 77 in the placebo group. In every study, the estimated survival curves started to diverge approximately after one year of treatment.

The 4S study population was updated after 2 years from the end of the study [22]. Subjects in the original statin group were reported as using cholesterol-lowering medication slightly more frequently, 85.5% vs 81.5% in the original placebo group. Of the placebo- and statin-treated subjects, 97 (4.9%) and 74 (3.6%) had died during the follow-up, suggesting that long-term treatment with statin up to 8 years was safe and the survival benefit still continued. It was expected that occurrence of malignancies had been higher in the original statin than in the original placebo group, owing to life prolongation in the former one. However, if anything, the death rate of malignancies tended to be reduced in the original statin group (p = 0.087).

Major coronary events

The relative risk of MCEs was constantly lower in the statin- than in the placebo-treated groups in all studies, such that the change in the relative risk of MCE was significantly lowered by statin from 24% to 34% (Tab. 1). In 4S, there were 622 (28%) MCEs in the placebo vs 431 (19%) in the statin group; in CARE the respective figures were 274 (13.2%) and 212 (10.2%). In primary prevention, the number of events was lower, such that in WOSCOPS, 248 (7.9%) MCEs occurred in the placebo and 174 (5.5%) in the statin group, and in AFCAPS/TexCAPS the respective figures were 183 (5.5%) and 116 (3.5%). Accordingly, in spite of different statins, study populations and baseline cholesterol values, the relative risk reduction of MCEs was of similar magnitude in the different studies. In every study, the probability curves of the statin and placebo groups for escaping MCE started to diverge from each other after approximately one year, and the diversion grew wider during the following years similarly to the survival curves. It is surprising that recurrence curves of coronary events of statin and placebo treatment do not differ until at the end of one year, even though the endothelial function improves much faster [1].

Statins lowered MCEs equally effectively in both sexes [9, 10, 12, 23], in elderly compared with younger subjects [9–12, 23], in type II diabetes and even in subjects with impaired fasting glucose levels [24, 25].

Other atherosclerotic manifestations

Statins reduced the need for hospitalization for unstable angina [10, 12], and the need for coronary bypass grafting or revascularization [8–12]. The number of fatal and/or nonfatal cerebrovascular events was significantly lower in the statin vs placebo group in 4S, CARE and LIPID, but the number of events was fairly low. However, it has been shown that a lowering of LDL cholesterol level by at least 25% prevents the progression of carotid artery intima and media thickening [15], an essential risk factor for stroke. Intermittent claudication appears to be significantly reduced by statin treatment; effective cholesterol lowering also prevents progression of atherosclerosis in lower leg arteries [16]. In type II diabetics and in subjects with impaired fasting glucose levels, the need for revascularization [25] and the number of any atherosclerotic events [24] were less frequent in the statin *vs* placebo groups. On the whole, any atherosclerosis-related end- point event was lower in the statin than in the placebo group, irrespective of age and sex [23]. In an elderly, 60–80 year old population, 3- to 5-year statin treatment significantly reduced ischemic cardiovascular events (cerebrovascular, ischemic heart and peripheral vascular diseases and sudden death), especially in diabetic subjects with a poor glucose control [17].

Major coronary events vs *serum lipids*

The results indicate that lowering serum cholesterol reduces the severity of coronary disease and regresses the atherosclerotic process, and the benefit of cholesterol lowering is considered incontrovertible. Which of the serum lipoprotein lipids were most important in this respect? It was obvious that if LDL cholesterol was not reduced, there was no risk reduction [26]. MCEs were reduced as effectively, regardless of the baseline LDL cholesterol level, indicating that statin was equally effective in subjects with low or high baseline LDL cholesterol level [9, 10, 21, 26]. On-treatment LDL cholesterol [19, 20] or apoprotein B level [21] was a significant predictor of the number of MCEs, indicating that the lower the LDL cholesterol level was at the end of the trial, the better the subjects' outcome was. The change in LDL cholesterol from baseline *per se* was associated with the reduction of MCE in 4S, but not in CARE.

The role of HDL cholesterol and serum triglycerides in coronary risk reduction was less consistent. In some [21, 26, 27], but not in all [18] studies, baseline HDL cholesterol was an important predictor of coronary risk as well as baseline serum triglyceride levels [26], but these associations were not evaluated using multivariate analysis.

In subgroup analyses, the decline in LDL cholesterol level was compared with the decrease in risk for MCEs. In 4S, the association was curvilinear, suggesting that greater LDL cholesterol reductions were followed by continuously decreasing reductions in coronary risk [19]. Similar results were obtained in AFCAPS/TexCAPS [21], whereas in CARE and LIPID, there was a threshold of LDL cholesterol value under which the rate of events was unchanged [9, 10, 20]. The threshold value of LDL cholesterol in LIPID was surprisingly high, 3.5 mmol/l, whereas in CARE the variation was wide-ranging from 3.2 mmol/l to 1.8 mmol/l. In WOSCOPS, a 24% fall in LDL cholesterol level was sufficient, and more aggressive LDL cholesterol reduction did not bring any more benefit [26]. The reason for the inconsistency of these results is not obvious, and National Cholesterol Education Program guidelines [28] for LDL cholesterol in secondary prevention <2.6 mmol/l and in primary prevention <3.0 mmol/l are considered well justified [14]. However, aggressive cholesterol lowering obtained with statin alone or combined with cholestyramine, delayed the progression of atheroscleroris in saphenous vein-coronary artery bypass grafts by 31%, irrespective of gender and age, and the presence of the most frequent coronary heart disease risk factors [29, 30]. The only variable differentiating the groups was on-treatment LDL cholesterol level, which in the treatment group was less than 2.5 mmol/l and in the placebo group 3.5 mmol/l, suggesting that even further LDL lowering than the recommended guidelines may turn out to be favourable to control atherosclerosis.

Other studies

After cardiac transplantation, pravastatin significantly reduced the serum cholesterol level of hypercholesterolemic patients, improved their survival and reduced the frequency of severe cardiac rejection and MCE [31]. In a recent study, the efficacy of aggressive cholesterol lowering with atorvastatin was compared with percutaneous coronary revascularization to reduce recurrences of coronary events in coronary subjects with an average LDL cholesterol level of 3 mmol/l [32]. After an 18-month follow-up, the number of ischemic events (including MCE, worsening of angina, angioplasty or coronary artery bypass grafting) was 36% lower in the statin than in the angioplasty group. LDL cholesterol was lowered by 1 mmol/l (about 28% reduction compared with the angioplasty group). This is a remarkable study, even though the study population was small and strictly selected, because these are the first results suggesting that by effective lowering of LDL cholesterol level the need for invasive coronary procedures can be controlled at least to some extent, which will have a large clinical and economical importance.

The statin trials have strengthened not only the cause-effect relationship between serum total and LDL cholesterol level and coronary artery disease, but also the causality that by lowering LDL cholesterol level the number of coronary events can be reduced and the progression of atherosclerosis in the whole vascular tree can be retarded or even ceased. These studies, however, give no information on non-responsiveness; it can be assumed that there are subjects in whom statins do not effectively lower LDL cholesterol level or, in spite of LDL cholesterol lowering, the statins do not reduce the recurrences of coronary events. An example of non-responsiveness is a recently reported possible genetic cause, a polymorphism in the gene coding cholesteryl ester transfer protein (CETP), affecting the progression of atherosclerosis [33]. CETP mediates the exchange of lipids between HDL and the other lipoproteins in the reverse cholesterol transport process. The presence of a specific polymorphism of the CETP gene (TaqIB) resulted in a lower HDL cholesterol level, higher plasma CETP concentration, and an association of progression of coronary atherosclerosis during a 2-year follow-up. In addition, pravastatin slowed the progression of coronary atherosclerosis, especially in those subjects having the polymorphism (B1B1), but not in those lacking it (B2B2). Pravastatin had similar effects on serum lipids in the different polymorphic groups, such that the progression was not related to serum lipid levels. Information on detailed mechanisms regulating an individual's responsiveness to lower serum cholesterol and to reduce recurrences of coronary events is of great clinical importance. Another example of non-responsiveness to statin-induced reduction of coronary events is high baseline absorption and low synthesis of cholesterol as presented in the following chapter.

Effects of statins on non-cholesterol sterols

From among the non-cholesterol sterols, found in small amounts in serum, precursor sterols, e.g., cholestenol, desmosterol and lathosterol, reflect cholesterol synthesis and especially its changes [34–38]. On the other hand, cholestanol and plant sterols, campesterol and sitosterol, are indicators of cholesterol absorption [37, 39, 40]. Since the statins inhibit cholesterol synthesis, the lowering of precursor sterol ratios to cholesterol may reflect this reduction, whereas it would be interesting to see responses of the sterols reflecting cholesterol absorption.

Short-term treatment

Statins were shown to decrease serum lathosterol contents during short-term treatment of hypercholesterolemia [38, 41–43], even in homozygous form of familial hypercholesterolemia (FH) [44]. Reduced precursor sterol levels were also related to decreased hepatic HMG-CoA reductase activity, despite a marked increase of the reductase protein content in human liver [43]. Statin-induced reduction of precursor sterol ratios were increased by combining bile acid binding agents, guar gum and resin treatments, back to baseline values or even above them, owing to enhanced cholesterol synthesis [41]. Pravastatin and lovastatin similarly reduced precursor sterol ratios at similar cholesterol lowering [45]. A closer analysis showed that both free and esterified serum lathosterol and other methylated and also demethylated precursor sterol ratios were decreased by a short-term pravastatin treatment in FH without and with an ileal by-pass operation [42]. Sterol balance data indicated that especially in the patients with ileal by-pass, both bile acid and cholesterol synthesis were decreased, and, in addition, both absolute and relative cholesterol absorption were reduced. Fecal output of precursor sterols was also reduced, but despite reduced cholesterol absorption, ratios of serum plant sterol to cholesterol tended to increase in serum [42].

Other short-term statin trials have also shown a tendency to increase or even significant elevations of serum cholestanol and plant sterol ratios [41, 45–49]. A combination of pravastatin with fibrate reduced the fibrate-induced increase of serum precursor sterols and increased the respective serum plant sterol ratios [48]. In addition, a combination of a small statin dose with plant stanol ester margarine consumption reduced the increased cholesterol synthesis caused by plant stanol esters, and further lowered serum cholesterol such that about 70% of postmenopausal coronary women reached the goal of LDL cholesterol <2.6 mmol/l [50]. A combination of plant stanol ester with statin further lowered cholesterol, increased precursor sterols and lowered cholesterol absorption markers [50–52].

Long-term treatment

Analysis of the non-cholesterol sterols in 4S patients of the Finnish subgroup showed that during the 5-year treatment period, the ratios of the serum precursor sterols to cholesterol were decreased by about 40% as compared with the pre-treatment or control values [53]. The respective values of the absorption indicators were increased by 10–20%. Explanation of the latter findings has been related to a possible decrease of biliary sterol secretion and a trend to increase absorption of these sterols from the reduced intestinal cholesterol pool. Owing to the rapid reduction of LDL cholesterol, shortly after the start of the statin treatment, the serum plant sterol concentrations decreased, whereas during the prolonged treatment, not only the ratio, but also the concentrations of plant sterols were increased in serum [54]. On the other hand, the marked reduction of the serum precursor sterol ratios can be related to high activity of the enzymes converting lanosterol to cholesterol in the presence of inhibited HMG-CoA reductase activity. Thus, the reduction of the serum precursor sterol ratios is higher than the absolute reduction of cholesterol synthesis measured by the sterol balance technique.

Division of the serum non-cholesterol sterols by baseline ratios of cholestanol to quartiles revealed that the 4S subjects with the highest baseline cholestanol quartile did not reduce recurrences of coronary events by the five-year simvastatin treatment as did those with the lowest respective quartile [55]. The subjects of the fourth quartile were considered to have high absorption and low synthesis of cholesterol, being accordingly less favourable for statin-induced lowering of cholesterol. The subjects of the first quartile with high serum precursor ratios had higher baseline synthesis of cholesterol and, accordingly, were ideal for statin-induced cholesterol lowering. The lowering of serum cholesterol was, actually, significantly less in the fourth than in the first quartile, yet the difference was relatively small, raising doubts as to whether it could be responsible for the difference in coronary events [54]. An additional observation was that the concentration of the plant sterols was gradually increased after an initial fall, especially in the fourth quartile in relation to the first one, such that the respective serum plant sterol ratio of LDL was markedly high in the fourth quartile at the end of the 5-year treatment. This raises the question of whether increased serum and lipoprotein plant sterols contributed to the absence of a reduction of coronary events in the fourth quartile.

The combination of cholesterol malabsorption caused by stanol ester consumption and statin-treated subjects further reduced serum LDL cholesterol, but also decreased elevated plant sterol levels [50, 51]. In fact, the decrease of plant sterols and LDL cholesterol caused by stanol ester margarine consumption was more consistent in statin-treated coronary patients with high rather than low baseline cholestanol ratio [52]. The findings suggest that statins and stanol ester combination may protect coronary patients with the high baseline cholestanol and plant sterol to cholesterol ratios from coronary recurrences.

Mean blood glucose decreased with increasing cholestanol and plant sterol ratios. However, a subgroup of patients with a high blood glucose and the high cholestanol ratio exhibited recurrent coronary events during the simvastatin treatment in the 4S [56]. In fact, the baseline glucose value was lower (4.77 ± 0.04 mmol/l) in subjects with a good response (LDL cholesterol <2.6 mmol/l) to simvastatin than in those (4.97 ± 0.04 mmol/l) with a less good response (LDL cholesterol > 2.6 mmol/l).

Effects of atorvastatin on serum non-cholesterol sterols

One-year statin treatment (20–40 mg/day) of coronary patients in the 3 T study lowered serum cholesterol slightly more effectively in the atorvastatin (–36%) than in the simvastatin (–32%) group [57]. The respective reductions of the serum precursor sterol ratios were also different (–50% vs –42%, respectively). However, the cholesterol absorption markers were markedly increased such that, e.g., the campesterol to cholesterol ratio was increased by about 82% *vs* 39% in the atorvastatin vs simvastatin group, the increment being highest in the third tertile defined by baseline serum cholestanol ratio. In contrast to the simvastatin treatment, the concentrations of serum sitosterol and campesterol also gradually increased by atorvastatin, one-year increments being about 10%, despite the marked reduction of their transporter lipoprotein LDL. This indicates, as in the five-year treatment of the 4S coronary patients [54], that during long-term atorvastatin treatment, the plant sterol contents of LDL particles gradually increase, suggesting that despite lowered LDL cholesterol concentration, the lipoprotein particles can transport increased amounts of plant sterols to arterial walls. It remains to be shown whether subjects with the highest baseline serum cholestanol and plant sterol tertiles will have unchanged recurrence of coronary events during long-term atorvastatin treatment, and whether the serum plant sterol values will get close to those seen in phytosterolemia. Measurement of non-cholesterol sterols during 80 mg/day of atorvastatin showed that, despite a dramatic reduction of cholesterol at 3 months of atorvastatin, the serum campesterol concentration had increased already by 2 mg/dl [57]. The change is markedly higher than that found in the 3 T study with simvastatin or a smaller atorvastatin dose, or in the 4S [54]. Simultaneous inhibition of sterol absorption by consumption of plant stanol esters appeared to prevent increase of serum plant sterols.

References

1 Maron DJ, Fazio S, Linton MRF (2000) Current perspectives on statins. *Circulation* 101: 207–213
2 Miettinen M, Turpeinen O, Karvonen MJ, Elosuo R, Paavilainen E (1972) Effect of cholesterol-lowering diet on mortality from coronary heart disease and other causes: a twelve-year clinical trial in men and women. *Lancet* 2: 835–838

3 Hjermann I, Holme I, Velve Byre K, Leren P (1981) Effect of diet and smoking intervention on the incidence of coronary heart disease. Report from the Oslo Study Group of a randomised trial in healthy men. *Lancet* 2: 1303–1310
4 Burr ML, Gilbert JF, Holliday RM, Elwood PC, Fehily AM, Rogers S, Sweetnam PM, Deadman NM (1989) Effects of changes in fat, fish, and References reinfarction trial (DART). *Lancet* 2: 757–761
5 de Lorgeril M, Salen P, Martin J-L, Monjaud I, Delaye J, Mamelle N (1999) Mediterranean diet, traditional risk factors, and the rate of cardiovascular complications after myocardial infarction. Final report of the Lyon Diet Heart Study. *Circulation* 99: 779–785
6 Lipid Research Clinics program (1984) The Lipid Research Clinics Coronary Primary Prevention Trial results. I. Reduction in incidence of coronary heart disease. *JAMA* 251: 351–364
7 Canner PL, Berge KG, Wenger NK, Stamler J, Friedmann L, Prineas RJ, Friedewald W (1986) Fifteen year mortality in coronary Drug Project patients: long-term benefit with niacin. *J Am Coll Cardiol* 8: 1245–1255
8 Scandinavian Simvastatin Survival Study Group (1994) Randomised trial of cholesterol lowering in 4444 patients with coronary heart disease: the Scandinavian Simvastatin Survival Study (4S). *Lancet* 344: 1383–1389
9 Sacks FM, Pfeffer MA, Moye LA, Rouleau JL, Rutherford JD, Cole TG, Brown L, Warnica JW, Arnold JMO, Wun C-C et al, for the Cholesterol and Recurrent Events Trial Investigators (1996) The effect of pravastatin on coronary events after myocardial infarction in patients with average cholesterol levels. *N Engl J Med* 335: 1001–1009
10 The Long-Term Intervention with Pravastatin in Ischaemic Disease (LIPID) Study Group (1998) Prevention of cardiovascular events and death with pravastatin in patients with coronary heart disease and a broad range of initial cholesterol levels. *N Engl J Med* 339: 1349–1357
11 Shepherd J, Cobbe SM, Ford I, Isles CG, Lorimer AR, Macfarlane PW, McKillop JH, Packard CJ, for the West of Scotland Coronary Prevention Study Group (1995) Prevention of coronary heart disease with pravastatin in men with hypercholesterolemia. *N Engl J Med* 333: 1301–1307
12 Downs JR, Clearfield M, Weis S, Whitney E, Shapiro DR, Beere PA, Langendorfer A, Stein EA, Kruyer W, Gotto Jr AM, for the AFCAPS/TexCAPS Research Group (1998) Primary prevention of acute coronary events with lovastatin in men and women with average cholesterol levels. Results of AFCAPS/TexCAPS. *JAMA* 279: 1615–1622
13 Knopp RH (1999) Drug treatment of lipid disorders. *N Engl J Med* 341: 498–511
14 Grundy SM (1998) Statin trials and goals of cholesterol-lowering therapy. *Circulation* 97: 1436–1439
15 McMahon S, Sharpe N, Gamble G, Hart H, Scott J, Simes J, White H (1998) Effects of lowering average or below-average cholesterol levels on the progression of carotid atherosclerosis. *Circulation* 97: 1784–1790
16 Pedersen TR, Kjekshus J, Pyörälä K, Olsson AG, Cook TJ, Musliner TA, Tobert JA, Haghfelt T (1998) Effect of simvastatin on ischemic signs and symptoms in the Scandinavian Simvastatin Survival Study (4S). *Am J Cardiol* 81: 333–335
17 Ishikawa T (1997) Reduction of cardiovascular events in the elderly by pravastatin (the PATE study): Significance of diabetes mellitus. *Atherosclerosis* 134: 173
18 Scandinavian Simvastatin Survival Study Group (1995) Baseline serum cholesterol and treatment effect in the Scandinavian Simvastatin Survival Study (4S). *Lancet* 345: 1274–1275
19 Pedersen TR, Olsson AG, Færgeman O, Kjekshus J, Wedel H, Berg K, Wilhelmsen L, Haghfelt T, Thorgeirsson G, Pyörälä K et al for The Scandinavian Simvastatin Survival Study Group (1998) Lipoprotein changes and reduction in the incidence of major coronary heart disease events in the Scandinavian Simvastatin Survival Study (4S). *Circulation* 97: 1453–1460
20 Sacks FM, Moyé LA, Davis BR, Cole TG, Rouleau JL, Nash DT, Pfeffer MA, Braunwald E (1998) Relationship between plasma LDL concentrations during treatment with pravastatin and recurrent coronary events in the Cholesterol and Recurrent Events Trial. *Circulation* 97: 1446–1452
21 Gotto Jr AM, Whitney E, Stein EA, Shapiro DR, Clearfield M, Weis S, Jou JY, Langendörfer A, Beere PA, Watson DJ et al (2000) Relation between baseline and on-treatment lipid parameters and first acute major coronary events in the Air Force/Texas Coronary Atherosclerosis Prevention Study (AFCAPS/TexCAPS). *Circulation* 101: 477–484
22 Pedersen TR, Wilhelmsen L, Færgeman O, Strandberg TE, Thorgeirsson G, Troedsson L, Kristianson J, Berg K, Cook TJ, Haghfelt T et al on behalf of the Scandinavian Simvastatin

Survival Study Group (2000) Follow-up study of patients randomized in the Scandinavian Simvastatin Survival Study (4S) of cholesterol lowering. *Am J Cardiol* 86: 257–262
23 Miettinen TA, Pyörälä K, Olsson AG, Musliner TA, Cook TJ, Færgeman O, Berg K, Pedersen T, Kjekshus J for the Scandinavian Simvastatin Study Group (1997) Cholesterol-lowering therapy in women and elderly patients with myocardial infarction or angina pectoris. Findings from the Scandinavian Simvastatin Survival Study (4S). *Circulation* 96: 4211–4218
24 Pyörälä K, Pedersen TR, Kjekshus J, Færgeman O, Olsson AG, Thorgeirsson G, the Scandinavian Simvastatin Survival Study (4S) group (1997) Cholesterol lowering with simvastatin improves prognosis of diabetic patients with coronary heart disease. A subgroup analysis of the Scandinavian Simvastatin Survival Study (4S). *Diabetes Care* 20: 614–620
25 Haffner SM, Alexander CM, Cook TJ, Boccuzzi SJ, Musliner TA, Pedersen TR, Kjekshus J, Pyörälä K, for the Scandinavian Simvastatin Survival Study Group (1999) Reduced coronary events in simvastatin-treated patients with coronary heart disease and diabetes or impaired fasting glucose levels. Subgroup analyses in the Scandinavian Simvastatin Survival Study. *Arch Intern Med* 159: 2661–2667
26 West of Scotland Coronary Prevention Study Group (1998) Influence of pravastatin and plasma lipids on clinical events in the West of Scotland Coronary Prevention Study (WOSCOPS). *Circulation* 97: 1440–1445
27 Pfeffer MA, Sacks FM, Moyé LA, East C, Goldman S, Nash DT, Rouleau JR, Rouleau JL, Sussex BA, Theroux P et al (1999) Influence of baseline lipids on effectiveness of pravastatin in the CARE trial. *J Am Coll Cardiol* 33: 125–130
28 Expert Panel on Detection, Evaluation and Treatment of High Blood Cholesterol in Adults (Adult Treatment Panel II) (1994) *Circulation* 89: 1329–1445
29 The Post Coronary Artery Bypass Graft Trial Investigators (1997) The effect of aggressive lowering of low-density lipoprotein cholesterol levels and low-dose anticoagulation on obstructive changes in saphenous-vein coronary-artery bypass grafts. *N Engl J Med* 336: 153–162
30 Campeau L, Hunninghake DB, Knatterud GL, White CW, Domanski M, Forman SA, Forrester JS, Geller NL, Gobel FL, Herd JA et al and Post CABG Trial Investigators (1999) Aggressive cholesterol lowering delays saphenous vein graft atherosclerosis in women, the elderly, and patients with associated risk factors. NHLBI Post Coronary Artery Bypass Graft Clinical Trial. *Circulation* 99: 3241–3247
31 Kobashigawa JA, Katznelson S, Laks H, Johnson JA, Yeatman L, Wang XM, Chia D, Terasaki PI, Sabad A, Cogert GA et al (1995) Effect of pravastatin on outcomes after cardiac transplantation. *N Engl J Med* 333: 621–627
32 Pitt B, Waters D, Brown WV, van Boven AJ, Schwartz L, Title LM, Eisenberg D, Shurzinske L, McCormick LS, for the Atorvastatin *versus* Revascularization Treatment Investigators (1999) Aggressive lipid-lowering therapy compared with angioplasty in stable coronary artery disease. *N Engl J Med* 341: 70–76
33 Kuivenhoven JA, Jukema JW, Zwinderman AH, de Knijff P, McPherson R, Bruschke AV, Lie KI, Kastelein JJ (1998) The role of a common variant of the cholesteryl ester transfer protein gene in the progression of coronary atheroscleroris. The Regression Growth Evaluation Statin Study Group. *N Engl J Med* 338: 86–93
34 Miettinen TA (1970) Detection of changes in human cholesterol metabolism. *Ann Clin Res* 2: 300–320
35 Miettinen TA (1981) Effects of bile acid feeding and depletion on plasma and biliary squalene, methyl sterols and lathosterol. *In*: G Paumgartner, A Stiehl, W Gerok (eds): *Bile Acids and Lipids*. MTP Press Ltd, Lancaster, 255–262
36 Björkhem I, Miettinen T, Reihnér E, Ewerth S, Angelin B, Einarsson K (1987) Correlation between serum levels of some cholesterol precursors and activity of HMG-CoA reductase in human liver. *J Lipid Res* 28: 1137–1143
37 Miettinen TA, Tilvis RS, Kesäniemi YA (1990) Serum plant sterols and cholesterol precursors reflect cholesterol absorption and synthesis in volunteers of a randomly selected male population. *Am J Epidemiol* 131: 20–31
38 Kempen HJM, Glatz JFC, Leuven JAG, van der Voort HA, Katan MB (1988) Serum lathosterol concentration is an indicator of whole-body cholesterol synthesis in humans. *J Lipid Res* 29: 1149–1155
39 Tilvis RS, Miettinen TA (1986) Serum plant sterols and their relation to cholesterol absorption. *Am J Clin Nutr* 43: 92–97

40 Miettinen TA, Tilvis RS, Kesäniemi YA (1989) Serum cholestanol and plant sterol levels in relation to cholesterol metabolism in middle-aged men. *Metabolism* 38: 136–140
41 Uusitupa MIJ, Miettinen TA, Happonen P, Ebeling T, Turtola H, Voutilainen E, Pyörälä K (1992) Lathosterol and other noncholesterol sterols during treatment of hypercholesterolemia with lovastatin alone and with cholestyramine or guar gum. *Arterioscler Thromb* 12: 807–813
42 Vanhanen H, Kesäniemi YA, Miettinen TA (1992) Pravastatin lowers cholesterol, cholesterol-precursor sterols, fecal steroids, and cholesterol absorption in man. *Metabolism* 41: 588–595
43 Reihner E, Rudling M, Ståhlberg D, Berglund L, Ewerth S, Björkhem I, Einarsson K, Angelin B (1990) Influence of pravastatin, a specific inhibitor of HMG-CoA reductase, on hepatic metabolism of cholesterol. *N Engl J Med* 323: 224–228
44 Miettinen TA (1990) Cholesterol metabolism during hypolipidemic treatment with inhibitors of cholesterol synthesis. *In*: C Crepaldi, A Tiengo, G Enzi (eds): *Diabetes, Obesity and Hyperlipidemias. IV.* Elsevier Science Publishers, Amsterdam, 139–144
45 Vanhanen H, Miettinen TA (1992) Pravastatin and lovastatin similarly reduce serum cholesterol and its precursor levels in familial hypercholesterolemia. *Eur J Clin Pharmacol* 42: 127–130
46 Miettinen TA, Tikkanen MJ, Helve E, Ojala J-P (1990) Inhibition of dietary cholesterol absorption during lovastatin (Mevinolin) treatment. *Drug Invest* 2 Suppl 2: 29–35
47 Miettinen TA (1991) Inhibition of cholesterol absorption by HMG-CoA reductase inhibitor. *Eur J Clin Pharmacol* 40:Suppl 1: S19-S21
48 Vanhanen HT, Miettinen TA (1995) Cholesterol absorption and synthesis during pravastatin, gemfibrozil and their combination. *Atherosclerosis* 115: 135–146
49 Gylling H, Miettinen TA (1996) The effects of inhibiting cholesterol synthesis and absorption on cholesterol and lipoprotein metabolism in hypercholesterolemic non-insulin dependent diabetic men. *J Lipid Res* 37: 1776–1785
50 Gylling H, Radhakrishnan R, Miettinen TA (1997) Reduction of serum cholesterol in postmenopausal women with previous myocardial infarction and cholesterol malabsorption induced by dietary sitostanol ester margarine. *Circulation* 96: 4226–4231
51 Vuorio A, Gylling H, Turtola H, Kontula K, Ketonen P, Miettinen TA (2000) Stanol ester margarine alone and with simvastatin lowers serum cholesterol in families with familial hypercholesterolemia caused by the FH- North Karelia mutation. *Arterioscler Thromb Vasc Biol* 20: 500–506
52 Gylling H, Miettinen TA (1998) Dietary stanol ester in statin-treated coronary patients with high basal cholesterol values. *Circulation* 98: Suppl I-585
53 Miettinen TA, Strandberg T, Vanhanen H, Gylling H, for the 4SGroup (1996) Non-cholesterol serum sterols in Scandinavian Simvastatin Survival Study. *In*: AM Gotto Jr, R Paoletti, LC Smith, AI Catapano, AS Jackson (eds): *Drugs affecting lipid metabolism. Risk factors and future directions.* Kluwer Academic Publishers, Dordrecht, *Medical Science Symposium series* 10: 473–476
54 Miettinen TA, Strandberg TE, Gylling H, for the Finnish Investigators of the Scandinavian Simvastatin Survival Study Group (2000) Noncholesterol sterols and cholesterol lowering by long-term simvastatin treatment in coronary patients. Relation to basal serum cholestanol. *Arterioscler Thromb Vasc Biol* 20: 1340–1346
55 Miettinen TA, Gylling H, Strandberg T, Sarna S, for the Finnish 4S Investigators (1998) Baseline serum cholestanol as predictor of recurrent coronary events in subgroup of Scandinavian simvastatin survival study. *BMJ* 316: 1127–1130
56 Miettinen TA, Gylling H (1998) Basal non-cholesterol sterols reveal a subgroup of 4S not benefitted by simvastatin-induced decrease of recurrent coronary events. *J Am Coll Cardiol* 31 Suppl A: 281A
57 Miettinen TA, Gylling H (2001) ABCG5/8 genes responsible for serum plant sterol increase during stativ treatment. XIV Intern Symp on Drugs Affecting Lipid Metabolism. New York, Abstract Book: 31

HMG-CoA Reductase Inhibitors
ed. by G. Schmitz and M. Torzewski

Cost-effectiveness of statins in primary and secondary prevention of coronary heart disease

Colin Berry[1], Andrew Davie[2] and John McMurray[1]

[1] *Department of Cardiology, Western Infirmary, Glasgow G11 6NT, Scotland, UK*
[2] *Southern General Hospital, 1345 Govan Road, Glasgow G51 4TF, Scotland, UK*

Introduction

Coronary heart disease (CHD) remains a major cause of ill health and premature death worldwide. As a result, healthcare costs for patients with CHD are substantial. Consequently, both the primary and secondary prevention of CHD are major objectives of healthcare systems worldwide. Recently, large, multicentre, clinical trials have demonstrated consistently that these objectives can be achieved though cholesterol-lowering therapy with 3-hydroxy-3-methyglutaryl coenzyme A reductase inhibitor (statin) therapy. In this article, we will first discuss the methods employed in cost-effectiveness analyses. Subsequently, we will review the cost-effectiveness of statin therapy in relation to different clinical trials undertaken for the primary and secondary prevention of CHD. Subsequently, the cost-effectiveness of statin therapy in other patient groups who were not included in these trials, such as the elderly, will also be considered. In addition, we will also consider the relative cost-effectiveness of different statin therapies. Finally, we will consider the cost-effectiveness of statin therapy and resource utilisation in relation to healthcare provision.

Component costs of healthcare expenditure on coronary heart disease

Coronary heart disease is characterised by impaired quality of life (QoL) [1], substantial morbidity and a high risk of premature death. Patients with these conditions also consume a substantial proportion of healthcare expenditure; however, the cost to society is even greater, because of the social and welfare costs involved (Tab. 1).

Methods of cost-effectiveness analysis

Economic evaluations of the cost of care include cost-effectiveness or cost minimisation analyses [2]. Cost-effectiveness evaluations typically use univer-

Table 1. The component costs of health-care expenditure on patients with coronary heart disease

Medical	Non-medical
Hospitalisation	Loss of income
Investigation	Carer support
Drug therapy	Welfare support
Ambulatory care (hospital outpatient/primary care)	Ambulance transport
Heart transplantation/CABG	

sal outcome measures, such as morbidity (e.g., hospitalisation rate) and mortality, for the evaluation of a treatment [3]. Such analyses typically incorporate direct costs (e.g., the costs of drug therapy, hospitalisation), but may also include an assessment of indirect costs (e.g., loss of income, welfare support). A cost-minimisation analysis may be used when a new treatment is associated with similar outcomes when compared with standard therapy. In this case the economic analysis simply evaluates which mode of treatment is cheaper.

There are several outcome units that may be used to measure the economic impact of different therapies. These include cost per life-year gained (LYG), cost per quality-adjusted life-year gained (QALY), and number needed to treat (NNT). The cost per LYG assesses the benefit of treatment purely in terms of mortality. This unit can be thought of as the cost required to extend one patient's life by one year. QALYs are a form of cost-utility analysis, which incorporate QoL information, expressed as a single index of utility (0–1), along with survival data. QALYs have become a standard measure in many economic analyses, although such application of QALYs is not universally supported [4]. NNT analysis, although not a direct measure of cost, is a strong predictor of cost-effectiveness. For a medical intervention, an NNT typically represents the number of individuals who need to be treated for a period of time (usually 5 years) to prevent the occurrence of one major morbid event. The smaller the NNT, the more likely the treatment is to be cost-effective.

Cost-effectiveness analyses may be undertaken on a prospective basis, where actual costs are quantified based on data collected during the clinical trial. Alternatively, cost-effectiveness analyses may be undertaken retrospectively, in which case clinical data from trials can be used to project costs in the context of a model. The Markov model is one such tool that is commonly used for cost-effectiveness analysis. This model assumes patients to be in one or more different health states. These may be simply alive or dead, or may range to several states ranging from health, disease (e.g., disease state A, or B, or C, etc.) in the presence or absence of a particular type of drug therapy [5]. The Markov model is an annual cycle process, in which all patients are assumed to 'transit' between health states, according to the probabilities of an event occurring, or lipid-lowering therapy being discontinued. These probability values can be obtained from data collected in randomised, controlled trials. The incremental costs for each cycle are calculated according to the number of patients in each health state. Total costs of therapy and effectiveness (e.g., life expectancy) can then be estimated by an iterative process for any future length of time.

Cost-effectiveness of statin therapy for the primary prevention of coronary heart disease

The West of Scotland coronary prevention study (WOSCOPS) randomised 6595 Scottish men aged 45–64 years with a total plasma cholesterol concentration of 7 ± 0.6 mmol/L (mean ± SD) and no evidence of previous myocardial infarction, to either placebo or pravastatin 40 mg/day, both in addition to dietary advice [6]. Medical records, electrocardiographic recordings, and the national death registry were used to determine the clinical end points. After an average of 4.9 years of follow-up, treatment with pravastatin was associated with reductions in plasma cholesterol concentrations by 20 percent and low-density lipoprotein cholesterol concentrations by 26 percent, compared with placebo. The annual risk of a cardiovascular event in this population was 1.5%. There were 248 definite coronary events (specified as nonfatal myocardial infarction or death from CHD) in the placebo group, and 174 in the pravastatin group (relative reduction in risk (RRR) with pravastatin, 31%; 95 percent confidence interval (95% CI), 17 to 43%; $p < 0.001$). There were similar reductions in the risk of definite nonfatal myocardial infarctions (31% reduction, $p < 0.001$), death from CHD (definite cases alone: 28% reduction, $p = 0.13$; definite plus suspected cases: 33% reduction, $p = 0.042$), and death from all cardiovascular causes (32% reduction, $p = 0.033$). Overall, a 22% reduction in the risk of death from any cause was observed in the pravastatin group (95% CI, 0 to 40 percent; $P = 0.051$). The results of this study have important implications for health-resource utilisation. In developed countries, where mortality rates from CHD are considerable, a relatively high proportion of the population also have an elevated plasma cholesterol concentration.

Caro et al. [7] undertook a cost-effectiveness analysis of the results of the WOSCOPS study. In this study, irreversible transition from health to disease (defined as the occurrence of either death or a cardiovascular event), was quantified on a monthly basis for 5 years, on an "intention to treat" basis. An estimate of life-years gained was made based on the difference between the age and sex-specific cumulative survival curves for Scotland [8], and the event-specific survival curves (these being derived from the Scottish Record Linkage System on 460,000 comparable cardiovascular events between 1981 and 1994. The costs of management of each type of event, for example, non-fatal myocardial infarction (MI), were estimated from extracontractual 1996 tariffs from a sample of 200 Scottish hospitals, with event-specific lengths of stay calculated from the WOSCOPS study. The cost of using pravastatin was £1.66 per 40 mg tablet per day. The costs of monitoring plasma chemistry for liver function and lipid profiles, and one visit to the general practitioner every 6 months, were also included. Indirect costs and costs incurred subsequent to the index event, were not included. Sensitivity analyses of the assumptions and uncertainties in this model were also carried out. The main outcome measures were the number of transitions from health to cardiovascular disease prevented, the number needed to treat (NNT) to prevent one transition event, and the cost per LYG.

For 10, 000 men started on pravastatin, 318 of them would be prevented from making the transition from health to cardiovascular disease (NNT 31.4), with a net cost-saving of £23,340,984 million ($36,449,280) over 5 years [7]. This equates to a cost-effectiveness ratio of £20,375 per LYG. This also equated to a saving of 2017 hospital-bed days saved. A sensitivity analysis of the lower limit of the 95% CI demonstrated that for a 12% reduction in death, the cost-effectiveness ratio is CI £15,068 to £37, 788 per LYG, whereas at the upper limit, a 33% reduction in death the cost-effectiveness ratio was between £5346 to £13, 419 per LYG. These figures were lower (£20,375; $31, 818) when calculations were repeated after a discount of 6% was made on all costs, as recommended by the United Kingdom Treasury. If the analysis is restricted to the 40% of men at highest risk, the NNT is reduced to 22.5 and the cost per LYG is £5601. The cost-effectiveness of pravastatin was estimated on a five-year basis; however, given that statin therapy is likely to be lifelong, and absolute risk increases with age, in this case, the cost-effectiveness of statin therapy may be underestimated.

These data compare very favourably with other healthcare interventions (Tab. 2), and suggest that lipid-lowering therapy should be considered for middle-aged men with elevated plasma cholesterol. Subgroup analyses in this study suggested that the cost-effectiveness was greater in patients at higher risk, such as those with additional risk factors for CHD.

The Airforce Coronary/Texas Coronary Atherosclerosis Prevention Study (AFCAPS/TexCAPs) was a randomised, double-blind, placebo-controlled trial of lovastatin for the prevention of a first acute major coronary event in both men and women without clinically evident atherosclerotic cardiovascular disease and who also had an average total cholesterol (TC) and LDL-C plasma concentration and below-average high-density lipoprotein cholesterol (HDL-C) plasma concentration [9]. A total of 5608 men and 997 women were included in this study. After an average follow-up of 5.2 years, lovastatin was associated with a reduction in the incidence of first acute major coronary events (183 vs 116 first events; relative risk [RR], 0.63; 95% confidence interval [CI], 0.50–0.79; $p < .001$), myocardial infarction (95 vs 57 myocardial infarctions; RR, 0.60; 95% CI, 0.43–0.83; $p = .002$), unstable angina (87 vs 60 first unstable angina events; RR, 0.68; 95% CI, 0.49–0.95; $p = .02$), coronary revascularization procedures (157 vs 106 procedures; RR, 0.67; 95% CI, 0.52–0.85; $P = .001$), coronary events (215 vs 163 coronary events; RR, 0.75;

Table 2. Assessment of the benefits of various cardiovascular treatments in terms of number needed to treat (NNT)

Treatment	Events prevented	NNT for 5 years to prevent 1 event
Antihypertensive therapy in elderly (STOP) [32]	Fatal and non-fatal cardiovascular events	6
Aspirin for TIA	Death, CVA	6
Warfarin for AF	CVA	7
ACE inhibitors for mild heart failure	Cardiovascular death, hospitalisation for CHF	8
Statin, post-MI (4S) trial [12]	CHD death, MI, cardiac arrest	10
Aspirin, post-MI	Cardiovascular death, MI, CVA	12
Statin, angina (4S trial) [12]	CHD death, MI, arrest	16
Antihypertensive therapy in elderly trial (SHEP trial) [33]	Fatal and non-fatal cardiovascular events	18
Statin, post-MI (CARE trial) [18]	CHD death, MI	33
Statin, asymptomatic men with raised LDL-C (WoSCoPS trial) [7]	CHD death, MI	31

TIA, transient ischaemic attack; AF, atrial fibrillation, CHD, coronary heart disease; CVA, cerebrovascular accident; ACE, angiotensin converting enzyme; CHF, congestive heart failure; MI, myocardial infarction; LDL-C, low-density lipoprotein cholesterol.

95% CI, 0.61–0.92; P = .006), and cardiovascular events (255 vs 194 cardiovascular events; RR, 0.75; 95% CI, 0.62–0.91; P = .003).

A cost-utilisation analysis of these results was conducted on prospectively collected data. As only direct medical costs were determined, this study was not a cost-effectiveness analysis [10]. Hospitalisation costs were calculated on the basis of diagnosis-related group (DRG) data and medical costs were calculated from the perspective of a private, single payer. Cardiovascular-related costs were calculated on the basis of 1996 MEDSTAT figures for the United States. The cost of lovastatin therapy in the United States in 1998 was also included in the analysis. Cardiovascular healthcare costs for the 5.2 years follow-up were, on average, $1931 for a placebo-treated patient and $1407 for a lovastatin-treated patient. This represents an 11% cost-saving on the total cost of lovastatin ($4,654) during this time period. This was the first study to provide information on costs and resource utilisation of primary prevention therapy with a statin in a low-risk population, which included women and elderly individuals.

Cost-effectiveness of statin therapy for the secondary prevention of coronary heart disease

The Scandinavian Simvastatin Survival Study (4S) was designed to evaluate the effect of cholesterol lowering with simvastatin on mortality and morbidity in patients with CHD [11]. This was a randomised, double-blind, placebo-controlled trial of cholesterol-lowering in 4444 patients with a history of angina pectoris or previous MI and a total serum cholesterol concentration of 5.5–8.0 mmol/L on a lipid-lowering diet. Over the 5.4 years median follow-up period, simvastatin therapy was associated with changes in total cholesterol, low-density-lipoprotein cholesterol, and high-density-lipoprotein cholesterol concentrations of –25%, –35%, and +80%, respectively. The relative risk of death in the simvastatin group was 0.70 (95% CI 0.58–0.85, p = 0.0003), such that the 6-year probabilities of survival in the placebo and simvastatin groups were 87.6% and 91.3%, respectively. There were 189 coronary deaths in the placebo group and 111 in the simvastatin group (relative risk 0.58, 95% CI 0.46–0.73). A coronary event occurred in 622 patients (28%) and 431 (19%) patients in the placebo and simvastatin groups, respectively. Other benefits of simvastatin therapy included a 37% reduction ($p < 0.00001$) in the risk of undergoing a myocardial revascularisation procedure. This study demonstrated that cholesterol-lowering therapy improves survival in CHD patients.

The impact of this intervention on the utilisation of healthcare resources was evaluated by Pedersen et al. [12]. This was a prospectively planned resource utilisation analysis based on information about the number of cardiovascular hospitalisations, length of stay, revascularisation procedures and concomitant medication usage. The costs of these hospitalisations were estimated by use of DRG MEDSTAT figures in the USA. The cost of drug therapy incorporated the costs for simvastatin (April 1995). A cost-minimisation analysis, extrapolated to the effects of simvastatin in the United States, demonstrated that over a 5.4-year period, costs associated with hospitalisation for cardiovascular disease would be reduced by 31%, or $3872 per patient. Overall, the DRG-based estimates of expenditure on acute hospitalisations and procedures for 100 patients during this time are $1.23 million, which represents 88% of the cost of simvastatin for the same patients. This could be an underestimate, as other costs, such as those for nursing-home care and indirect costs (e.g., loss of income), were not included in this analysis.

The cost-effectiveness of simvastatin as a secondary prevention measure was also explored by Jonsson et al. [13]. A Markov model was used in which two cohorts, one receiving usual therapy and the other taking statin therapy, were 'tracked', with outcomes and costs quantified for both groups. This differed from the reference model inasmuch as all states were disease-related. The model used data from 4S for males and females aged 35 to 64 years, and 65 years and older, who had a maximum possible survival of 110 years. The probability of a coronary event, or death, was then determined. The study incorporated both direct and indirect costs based on costs of healthcare utilisation and salaries in Sweden in 1995. Adjustment for QoL was not performed.

The cost per LYG for treatment with simvastatin over a 5-year period ranged from $3,800 to $27,400 [13]. If indirect costs are also included, then the cost per LYG ranged from $1,200 to $13,300. The cost per LYG is increased in females and the elderly. For example, the cost per LYG in a 59-year-old male, whose total plasma cholesterol concentration was 261 mg/dL (6.8 mmol/L), was $5,400, or $1,600 if indirect costs are included. The costs in a woman of the same age were $10,500 and $5,100, respectively. If these data are applied to other healthcare systems, such as the UK, the cost per LYG would be £5502 [13].

These data compare favourably with a cost analysis for lovastatin as a secondary prevention intervention [14]. In this analysis, which used data from epidemiological studies rather than data from randomised trials, treatment with 20 mg of lovastatin per day, compared to usual care, was associated with a cost-effectiveness ratio of $9400 to $30,000 per life-year saved (1989 US$). Clearly, the cost-effectiveness of these therapies is affected by the patient's age, sex and plasma cholesterol concentration, all of which contribute to the patient's absolute risk of a future ischaemic event. Taken together, these data demonstrate that secondary prevention with statin therapy can be extremely cost-effective in certain groups of patients.

Analyses performed in the North of England Evidence-based Guidelines Development Project found that treating 1000 patients who have experienced an MI with a statin for one year will avoid 4 deaths (95% CI: 2 to 6 deaths). Additionally, 6 non-fatal MIs (95% CI: 2 to 10) and two non-fatal strokes (95% CI: 1 to 3) will be avoided [15]. In England and Wales, secondary prevention with simvastatin is now indicated in patients post-MI with a plasma cholesterol concentration of >5.4 mmol/L [16].

Cost-effectiveness of cholesterol lowering in other patient groups

Secondary prevention in the elderly

One limitation of large, randomised, controlled trials is their exclusion of certain groups of patients, such as the elderly. In 4S, patients aged >70 years were excluded from the study. In the CARE study, however, participants aged 65–75 years had comparable benefits from lipid-lowering therapy, compared to the effect of treatment in the study as a whole.

Ganz et al. [17] sought to determine whether or not secondary prevention with lipid-lowering therapy might also be cost-effective in the elderly. They used a Markov model to estimate the cost-effectiveness of statin therapy in a hypothetical group of elderly patients, aged 75–84 years, with a history of MI, using results from this age-group in published randomised-controlled trials. In this study, follow-up data from the CARE trial [18] were used to estimate the RRR conferred by statin therapy for MI (non-fatal and fatal combined) and stroke patients aged 65–75 years of age. It should be noted that these data are estimates of treatment effect in this age group and, as such, are not strictly evidence-based. The model did not allow for recurrent or multiple events; other health states, such as chronic heart failure, were not included in the model, but were incorporated into mortality estimates and QoL. In their sensitivity analysis, the effects of drug therapy were limited to 5 years. In this case, patients on statin therapy are modelled to have the same event rates as those on placebo, such that a conservative estimate can be made, in which case the drug has no additional effects beyond the duration of the clinical trial. Healthcare utilisation costs were estimated based on 1998 Medicare charges, the 1999 Ernst and Young Diagnosis-Related Group Handbook for the fiscal year 1997 and the cost of institutional care after stroke was estimated based on data from GUSTO-I. The cost of 40 mg of pravastatin per day was also included in the analysis.

In the base-case analysis, the incremental cost-effectiveness of statin therapy for the prevention of MI, compared with usual care, in patients 75–84 years of age with a previous MI was $18,800 per QALY. In the sensitivity analysis, the cost-effectiveness ratio for protection against fatal and non-fatal MI ranged from $12,100 to $77,500, whereas the cost-effectiveness of statin therapy for stroke prevention in these patients was $16,200 to $24,000. These data compare favourably with one other cost-effectiveness analysis of statin therapy in the elderly [14]. These data suggest that secondary prevention with statin therapy in the elderly can be a cost-effective measure, compared with the cost-effectiveness of other medical interventions (Tab. 2).

Primary and secondary prevention of cardiovascular events in different risk groups

The cost-effectiveness of statin therapy is a function of both the patient's absolute risk and the cost of the drug therapy. Absolute risk is determined by factors such as, age, sex, past medical history and the presence of risk factors for CHD, including plasma cholesterol concentration. Prosser et al. [19] set out to quantify how cost-effectiveness varies according to the presence or absence of these factors. They used the Coronary Heart Disease Policy Model, which is a previously validated cost-effectiveness instrument [20]. QoL parameters were ascribed according to the Beaver Dam Health Outcomes Study [21]. Costs were based on the Medical Care Component of the Consumer Price Index (US$ 1997). They found that cost-effectiveness ratios for primary prevention ranged from $54,000 to $420,000 per QALY for men and from $62,000 to $1,400,000 for women. These ratios were generally less than $100,000 for men and women (except women <45 years) with one or more risk factors for CHD. Interestingly, these ratios were affected not just by the number of risk factors present, but also their type of combination. In terms of secondary prevention, cost-effectiveness ratios were less than $50,000 per QALY for all subgroups, and were cost-saving for several subgroups for men with one or more risk factor [19]. These data suggest that primary prevention in young men and women, particularly in those without risk factors, may not be cost-effective, whereas secondary prevention is almost universally cost-effective.

Cost-effectiveness of different statins

The lipid-lowering potency and cost of different statins varies widely. Furthermore, the evidence base in support of the use of this class of drug is different for each individual drug. These factors therefore present a problem to clinicians and healthcare providers as to which statin should be prescribed for different patients. Huse et al. [22] addressed this problem in one recent study which used a decision-analytic model based on findings obtained from a Markov model. For drug therapy, the usual starting doses of the different statins were used (atorvastatin 10 mg, fluvastatin 20 mg, lovastatin 20 mg, pravastatin 20 mg, or simvastatin 10 mg), or no drug therapy at all. The effects of these statins on plasma lipids were estimated from approved US Food and Drug Administration product labelling [23]. Annual mortality rates from CHD and healthcare costs were estimated from information collected in the Framingham study [24]. Costs and life-expectancy were discounted at an annual rate of 3%. Atorvastatin was found to be the most cost-effective statin, compared to no drug therapy, for either primary prevention or secondary prevention [22]. The limitations of this study include the lack of prospective data, and the applicability of these findings to populations other than white, middle-aged, middle-class subjects, which predominate in the town of Framingham.

Health economics of the treatment of hyperlipidaemia

Patients with CHD are at high risk of further morbid events. This can be associated with considerable use of healthcare resources, resulting in substantial consumption of healthcare expenditure. For example, in 1996, the total cost of CHD to the National Health Service and social care system in the United Kingdom was £1.63 billion [25]. The contribution of hypercholesterolaemia, as a risk factor for CHD, is estimated to represent 46% of total healthcare expenditure on CHD. If treatment of hypercholesterolaemia was associated with an overall reduction in blood cholesterol concentrations to less than 6.5 mmol/L, a 10% reduction in CHD events might be achieved [26].

At what level might a healthcare system consider an intervention to be cost-effective? An example of an intervention with a generally accepted level of cost-effectiveness is haemodialysis for patients with end-stage renal failure. The cost of this is approximately £26,500 per QALY. In this context, secondary prevention with lipid-lowering therapy represents £5000 to £10,000 per QALY, and is, therefore, cost-effective. It is estimated that in England, 930,000 patients might benefit from statin therapy for the secondary prevention of CHD [27]. In this case, the potential cost-effectiveness of secondary prevention with statins is therefore limited by the underprescription of these drugs.

The case for primary prevention with lipid-lowering therapy, however, is less obvious. In WOSCOPS, treatment with pravastatin was beneficial in patients with a CHD event rate of 1.5% per annum. In this case, however, the NNT of 40 would equate to approximately 3.8 million people who could benefit from this treatment in the United Kingdom [27]. The European Joint Committee's recommendations to treat patients with a CHD risk of >2% per annum would equate of a NNT of 22.5, based on WOSCOPS. In this case, the cost per LYG would be £14,000 [7, 28]. Nevertheless, the cost implications of primary prevention are considerable. Clearly, the cost-effectiveness of primary prevention with statin therapy varies widely and is dependent on whether absolute risk is considered according to either the plasma cholesterol concentration alone, or absolute CHD risk. The latter is a function of factors such as a patient's age, sex, and the presence of other risk factors for CHD, and is a more comprehensive and accurate assessment of absolute risk [29, 30].

Pickin et al. [31] investigated the relationship between level of CHD risk, the cost of statin, and the cost-effectiveness of statin therapy. The levels of CHD risk per annum were: CHD risk of 4.5% per year (secondary prevention); and primary prevention at CHD risk levels of 3%, 2% and 1.5% per year. These CHD event rates reflect those of the placebo groups in 4S (CHD event rate of 4.5%) and WOSCOPS (CHD event rate of 1.5%). Drug costs were obtained from the British National Formulary (1997) and calculations were based on life-long therapy, with a 6% discount rate. Estimates of healthcare costs were based on National Health Service figures for the North East of England. The costs per LYG according to annual CHD event risk were for 4.5%, £5100; 3%, £8200; 2%, £10,700; and 1.5%, £12,500. The annual cost of statin treatment was also a major determinant of the cost-effectiveness of this intervention.

Treatment of patients on the basis of CHD risk, rather than concentration of plasma cholesterol, is therefore a more cost-effective and clinically relevant basis for treatment. Primary prevention therapy with statins for patients with a CHD risk of 1.5% per annum is clearly less cost-effective than therapy in patients at higher levels of absolute risk. However, these figures may prove less expensive in other countries with higher rates of intervention, such as in the USA, where the potential for cost saving with lipid-lowering therapy may be greater.

The question, in terms of primary prevention, is, therefore, who should be treated? At a population level, this question is best addressed with a treatment policy to guide both healthcare providers and clinicians. This treatment framework should incorporate a number of parameters, such as cost per LYG, QALY and NNT. Pickin et al. [31] argued that primary prevention with lipid-lowering therapy should be initiated in patients with an annual CHD risk of 3%, and this is the current basis for primary prevention with lipid-lowering therapy in Scotland. Clearly, this level will exclude many patients who might otherwise have received a statin, and who may well subsequently develop CHD. Consequently, there is currently considerable debate with regard to the threshold. We share the view of Shepherd [28] that a more appropriate and cost-effective level for intervention with statins for the primary prevention of CHD would be in individuals with a greater than 2% annual risk [28].

References

1 Ware JE, Bayliss MS, Rogers WH, Kosinski M, Tarlov AR (1996) Differences in 4-year health outcomes for elderly and poor, chronically ill patients treated in HMO and fee-for-service systems – Results from the medical outcomes study. *JAMA* 276: 1039–1047

2 Drummond M, Torrance G, Mason J (1993) Cost-effectiveness league tables – more harm than good. *Soc Sci Med* 37: 33–40

3 Fletcher A (1991) Pressure to treat and pressure to cost – a review of cost- effectiveness analysis. *J Hypertens* 9: 193–198

4 Lapuma J, Lawlor EF (1990) Quality-adjusted life-years – ethical implications for physicians and policy-makers. *JAMA* 263: 2917–2921

5 Sonnenberg FA, Beck JR (1993) Markov models in medical decision making: a practical guide. *Med Decis Making* 13: 322–338

6 Shepherd J, Cobbe SM, Ford I, Isles CG, Lorimer AR, MacFarlane PW, McKillop JH, Packard CJ (1995) Prevention of coronary heart-disease with pravastatin in men with hypercholesterolemia. *N Engl J Med* 333: 1301–1307

7 Caro J, Klittich W, McGuire A, Ford J, Norrie J, Pettitt D, McMurray J, Shepherd J (1997) The west of Scotland coronary prevention study: economic benefit analysis of primary prevention with pravastatin. *BMJ* 315: 1577–1582

8 Registrar General Scotland (1995) Annual Report 1994. Her Majesty's Stationery Office, Edinburgh

9 Downs JR, Clearfield M, Weis S, Whitney E, Shapiro DR, Beere PA, Langendorfer A, Stein EA, Kruyer W, Gotto AM (1998) Primary prevention of acute coronary events with lovastatin in men and women with average cholesterol levels – Results of AFCAPS/TexCAPS. *JAMA* 279: 1615–1622
10 Gotto AM, Boccuzzi SJ, Cook JR, Alexander CM, Roehm JB, Meyer GS, Clearfield M, Weis S (2000) Effect of lovastatin on cardiovascular resource utilization and costs in the Airforce Coronary/Texas Coronary Atherosclerosis Prevention Study (AFCAPS/TexCAPs). *Am J Cardiol* 86: 1176–1181
11 Pedersen TR, Kjekshus J, Berg K, Haghfelt T, Faergeman O, Thorgeirsson G, Pyorala K, Miettinen T et al (1994) Randomized trial of cholesterol-lowering in 4444 patients with coronary-heart-disease – the Scandinavian Simvastatin Survival Study (4S). *Lancet* 344: 1383–1389
12 Pedersen TR, Kjekshus J, Berg K, Olsson AG, Wilhelmsen L, Wedel H, Pyorala K (1996) Cholesterol lowering and the use of healthcare resources – Results of the Scandinavian Simvastatin Survival Study. *Circulation* 93: 1796–1802
13 Jonsson B, Johannesson M, Kjekshus J, Olsson AG, Pedersen TR, Wedel H (1996) Cost-effectiveness of cholesterol lowering – Results from the Scandinavian Simvastatin Survival Study (4S). *Eur Heart J* 17: 1001–1007
14 Goldman L, Weinstein MC, Goldman PA, Williams LW (1991) Cost-effectiveness of HMG-COA reductase inhibition for primary and secondary prevention of coronary heart-disease. *JAMA* 265: 1145–1151
15 North of England Evidence-based Guidelines Development Project (2001) Prophylaxis for patients who have experienced a myocardial infarction: drug treatment, cardiac rehabilitation and dietary manipulation. Department of Health, London, UK, 1–115
16 Guideline Development Group (2001) Prophylaxis for patients who have experienced a myocardial infarction. National Institute for Clinical Excellence, London, UK
17 Ganz DA, Kuntz KM, Jacobson GA, Avorn J (2000) Cost-effectiveness of 3-hydroxy-3-methylglutaryl coenzyme A reductase inhibitor therapy in older patients with myocardial infarction. *Ann Intern Med* 132: 780–787
18 Lewis SJ, Moye LA, Sacks FM, Johnstone DE, Timmis G, Mitchell J, Limacher M, Kell S, Glasser SP, Grant J et al (1998) Effect of pravastatin on cardiovascular events in older patients with myocardial infarction and cholesterol levels in the average range – Results of the cholesterol and recurrent events (CARE) trial. *Ann Intern Med* 129: 681–686
19 Prosser LA, Stinnett AA, Goldman PA, Williams LW, Hunink MGM, Goldman L, Weinstein MC. (2000) Cost-effectiveness of cholesterol-lowering therapies according to selected patient characteristics. *Ann Intern Med* 132: 769–779
20 Weinstein MC, Coxson PG, Williams LW, Pass TM, Stason WB, Goldman L (1987) Forecasting coronary heart-disease incidence, mortality, and cost – the coronary heart-disease policy model. *Am J Public Health* 77: 1417–1426
21 Fryback DG, Dasbach EJ, Klein R, Klein BE, Dorn N, Peterson K, Martin PA (1993) The beaver dam health outcomes study – initial catalog of health-state quality factors. *Med Decis Making* 13: 89–102
22 Huse DM, Russell MW, Miller JD, Kraemer DF, D'Agostino RB, Ellison RC, Hartz SC (1998) Cost-effectiveness of statins. *Am J Cardiol* 82: 1357–1363
23 Physicians' Desk Reference (1998) Montvale, New Jersey
24 Russell MW, Huse DM, Drowns S, Hamel EC, Hartz SC (1998) Direct medical costs of coronary artery disease in the United States. *Am J Cardiol* 81: 1110–1115
25 Coronary Heart Disease Statistics (1998) British Heart Foundation. Economics Supplement, London
26 Britton A, McPherson K (2000) Monitoring the progress of the 2010 target for coronary heart disease mortality: estimated consequences on CHD incidence and mortality from changing prevalence of risk factors. National Heart Forum, London
27 Haq IU, Ramsay LE, Pickin DM, Yeo WW, Jackson PR, Payne JN (1996) Lipid-lowering for prevention of coronary heart disease: what policy now? *Clin Sci* 91: 399–413
28 Shepherd J (2001) Economics of lipid lowering in primary prevention: Lessons from the West of Scotland Coronary Prevention Study. *Am J Cardiol* 87(5A): 19B–22B
29 Haq IU, Jackson PR, Yeo WW, Ramsay LE (1995) Sheffield risk and treatment table for cholesterol-lowering for primary prevention of coronary heart-disease. *Lancet* 346: 1467–1471
30 Ramsay LE, Haq IU, Jackson PR, Yeo WW (1996) Targeting lipid-lowering drug therapy for pri-

mary prevention of coronary heart disease: An updated Sheffield table (vol 348, pg 387, 1996). *Lancet* 348: 1251–1252

31 Pickin DM, McCabe CJ, Ramsay LE, Payne N, Haq IU, Yeo WW, Jackson PR (1999) Cost effectiveness of HMG-CoA reductase inhibitor (statin) treatment related to the risk of coronary heart disease and cost of drug treatment. *Heart* 82: 325–332

32 Dahlof B, Hansson L, Lindholm L, Rastam L, Schersten B, Wester PO (1986) Stop-hypertension – Swedish trial in old patients with hypertension. *J Hypertens* 4: 511–513

33 Hulley SB, Furberg CD, Gurland B, McDonald R, Perry HM, Schnaper HW, Schoenberger JA, Smith WM, Vogt TM (1985) Systolic hypertension in the elderly program (SHEP) – antihypertensive efficacy of chlorthalidone. *Am J Cardiol* 56: 913–920

Index

MIX
Papier aus verantwortungsvollen Quellen
Paper from responsible sources
FSC® C105338

If you have any concerns about our products,
you can contact us on
ProductSafety@springernature.com

In case Publisher is established outside the EU,
the EU authorized representative is:
Springer Nature Customer Service Center GmbH
Europaplatz 3, 69115 Heidelberg, Germany

Printed by Libri Plureos GmbH
in Hamburg, Germany